"*The Big Book of Exposures* is a cornucopia of creative and effective exposure strategies for a range of anxiety disorders. The authors have cataloged hundreds of simple and effective exposures that they've tested in their own clinical practices. The exposures worked for them, and will work for you. If you're in search of thoughtful guidance on designing and implementing exposures, add this book to your bookshelf. You won't regret it."

> —**Michael A. Tompkins, PhD, ABPP**, codirector of the San Francisco Bay Area Center for Cognitive Therapy; assistant clinical professor at the University of California, Berkeley; and author of *Anxiety and Avoidance*

"Exposure therapy—helping patients therapeutically face their fears—is the most effective intervention for treating clinical fear and anxiety, and Springer and Tolin have amassed a comprehensive, practical guide to using this technique. Complete with loads of creative exposure ideas and suggestions, this book is a must for any clinician working with anxious and fearful individuals."

> —**Jonathan S. Abramowitz, PhD,** professor of psychology at The University of North Carolina at Chapel Hill, and author of *Getting Over OCD*

"Drawing from their extensive clinical experience and research expertise, Springer and Tolin have created an invaluable resource for both beginner and advanced clinicians who use, or who would like to use, exposure therapy in their practice. This practical guide is packed with evidence-informed, innovative recommendations for designing in vivo, interoceptive, and imaginal exposures for children and adults with a range of anxiety and related disorders. A 'must-read' for clinicians looking to expand their repertoire of clinical skills."

> —**Susan M. Orsillo, PhD**, professor of psychology at Suffolk University, and coauthor of *The Mindful Way through Anxiety*

"Confronting feared situations is among the most powerful approaches to treating anxiety and related disorders. This well-written, accessible book is filled with practical tips for conducting exposure therapy for the most common anxiety-related problems. This book will even help therapists to overcome their own apprehension about using exposure therapy, by addressing frequently occurring misconceptions and myths concerning exposure. *The Big Book of Exposures* is essential reading for any therapist who treats anxiety disorders, obsessive-compulsive disorder (OCD), post-traumatic stress disorder (PTSD), illness anxiety, and related problems—whether they are a student, novice clinician, or seasoned therapist."

> —**Martin M. Antony, PhD, ABPP**, professor of psychology at Ryerson University, and coauthor of *The Shyness and Social Anxiety Workbook* and *The Anti-Anxiety Workbook*

# THE
# BIG BOOK
## *of*
# EXPOSURES

## Innovative, Creative & Effective CBT-Based Exposures for Treating Anxiety-Related Disorders

### KRISTEN S. SPRINGER, PHD
### DAVID F. TOLIN, PHD

New Harbinger Publications, Inc.

## Publisher's Note

NEW HARBINGER PUBLICATIONS is a registered trademark of New Harbinger Publications, Inc.

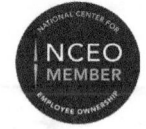

New Harbinger Publications is an employee-owned company.

Copyright © 2020 by Kristen S. Springer and David F. Tolin
New Harbinger Publications, Inc.
5720 Shattuck Avenue
Oakland, CA 94609
www.newharbinger.com

Cover design by Amy Shoup

Acquired by Tesilya Hanauer

Edited by Rona Bernstein

Indexed by James Minkin

---

Library of Congress Cataloging-in-Publication Data on file

Printed in the United States of America

26    25    24

10    9    8    7    6

*To my husband, Mike, who always said I would write a book. I never believed him. This one is for you.*—KSS

*To Fiona, James, and Katie, and to all of the clients who have taught me over the years.*—DFT

# Contents

# Introduction

*I learned that courage was not the absence of fear, but the triumph over it. The brave man is not he who does not feel afraid, but he who conquers that fear.*

—Nelson Mandela

As clinical psychologists who specialize in, and conduct research on, anxiety and related disorders, we have been using cognitive behavioral therapy (CBT) in our work to effectively treat hundreds of clients with a range of disorders, such as phobias, panic disorder, obsessive-compulsive disorder (OCD), posttraumatic stress disorder (PTSD), and more. Our aim in writing this book is to help you use a critical, yet underutilized, element of CBT for anxiety and related disorders: *exposure*. In this book, we have compiled hundreds of exposures that we have used with clients. From our many experiences using exposure in clinical settings, we have learned both the basics and the finer points of this intervention. And we have taught many other clinicians what we know about taking appropriate risks with exposures and getting creative with exposures to help clients target their core fears and get the most out of treatment.

That being said, we also get stuck from time to time on how to best design and implement an exposure for a particular client. That is what led to the development of this book. If we need ideas for exposure, then we imagine that so do many others who may not be using exposures regularly in their work. Therefore, we have created this book as an easy-to-use and up-to-date guide—using criteria from the *Diagnostic and Statistical Manual of Mental Disorders* (5th ed.; *DSM-5*; American Psychiatric Association [APA], 2013)—with nearly 400 exposures for you to flip through and find the best ones to suit each client.

## WHO THIS BOOK IS FOR

This book is primarily written for behavioral health professionals and trainees in behavioral health disciplines. We hope that whether you are a psychologist, social worker, mental health counselor, psychiatrist, or student in training to become one of these professionals, this book will be helpful for you in your treatment of clients with anxiety-related problems. The exposures in this book can be used to treat a range of clients in a variety of settings, such as an outpatient mental health clinic, a private practice setting, a school setting, or an inpatient unit. We have designed this book to be helpful to clinicians working with both younger and older client populations. Additionally, for ease of reading, throughout this book we alternate between using male and female pronouns in each chapter, but of course, regardless of the pronoun we use, the exposures are suitable for clients of any gender.

# HOW TO USE THIS BOOK

Part 1, "An Overview of Exposure Therapy," is designed to provide you with information about the empirical support for exposure with clients with panic, anxiety, phobias, OCD, and trauma-related disorders. We discuss common misconceptions that mental health providers may have about exposure work, aiming to help you solidify your rationale for using it as a treatment of choice for various anxiety-related disorders. We provide information and clinical vignettes to help you better engage fearful clients and to help them get on board with treatment. The mere idea of exposure therapy can make some clients (and clinicians) nervous or uncertain about what will take place and how it will go. Therefore, we aim to help you overcome any barriers that might be in your way as you move forward with delivering exposure therapy to your clients by outlining why it is safe and effective to use this in your work with clients. We also include a chapter dedicated to the nuances of doing successful exposure work with children and adolescents.

Part 2, "Getting Creative with Exposures for Anxiety and Related Disorders," gets into the diverse work that can be done with exposures. And, as you'll see, it really is fun work—creative, empowering, flexible, and, best of all, effective. We dedicate full chapters to each of the anxiety-related disorders for which you will commonly use exposure as a central component of treatment. These include specific phobias, panic disorder and agoraphobia, social anxiety disorder, OCD, acute stress disorder and PTSD, illness anxiety disorder, and separation anxiety disorder. Each chapter in part 2 includes many innovative exposure ideas for you to use to best match your clients' needs. In addition to the exposure examples, each of the chapters in part 2 contains resources such as imaginal scripts to use or adapt, games to play with your clients to target their fears, and more. These resources, as well as some from earlier chapters, are also available on the website dedicated to this book, http://www.newharbinger.com/43737, and can be downloaded, printed, and used with your clients. (See the very back of this book for more details.)

We hope that you find the guidance and instruction in this book helpful in learning not only how to use exposures successfully with your clients, but also how to get creative with designing your own unique exposures and implementing them with confidence.

# PART I

# An Overview of Exposure Therapy

# CHAPTER 1

# Anxiety, Avoidance, and Exposure

Anxiety disorders are the most common mental disorders, substantially exceeding the rate of depression, substance use disorders, and other conditions. In fact, nearly one third of Americans have a lifetime history of one or more anxiety disorders (Kessler, Petukhova, Sampson, Zaslavsky, & Wittchen, 2012). Therefore, it is important to disseminate effective treatments for anxiety to behavioral health providers. In this chapter, we will discuss the negative impact of anxiety, the factors that contribute to the development and maintenance of anxiety, and how to treat anxiety using exposure therapy.

## THE COST OF ANXIETY

Anxiety disorders are associated with significant functional, social, and economic burden. DuPont et al. (1996) estimated that the total cost of anxiety-related disorders was $46.6 billion in 1990, or 31.5% of the total economic burden of mental illness. Anxiety-related disorders are also associated with significant reductions in health-related quality of life (QOL) in the general population (Comer et al., 2011), in outpatient mental health settings (Lochner et al., 2003), and in primary care medical settings (Beard, Weisberg, & Keller, 2010). Across studies, individuals with anxiety disorders report much poorer QOL than do control participants, and this appears to be true across diagnoses (Olatunji, Cisler, & Tolin, 2007).

In addition to the burden of anxiety-related disorders on the individual, these disorders often have a significant negative impact on families. For example, family members of clients with OCD and PTSD report levels of distress, impairment, and burden comparable to those reported by family members of patients with schizophrenia (Kalra, Kamath, Trivedi, & Janca, 2008; Veltro, Magliano, Lobrace, Morosini, & Maj, 1994). There are also high levels of distress in intimate relationships (Cooper, 1996; Jordan et al., 1992; Riggs, Byrne, Weathers, & Litz, 1998). Family members often become ensnared in ritualistic or avoidant behaviors at the insistence of the client, which can be time-consuming and frustrating. In addition, the emotional and behavioral aspects of anxiety are associated with significant financial strain, disruption of family activities, and impaired family interactions (Black, Gaffney, Schlosser, & Gabel, 1998; Calvocoressi et al., 1995; Van Noppen & Steketee, 2003; Verbosky & Ryan, 1988). For these reasons, we often include family members in the treatment of anxiety-related disorders, especially when working with children and adolescents, an issue that we will address in chapter 4.

# WHAT IS ANXIETY?

Anxiety disorders can be conceptualized as an exaggerated pattern of fearful responding that has a negative impact on the individual's life. Fear is composed of physiological, cognitive, and behavioral elements, which we will discuss below.

## Anxiety and Physiology

Physiologically, fear is associated with sympathetic nervous system activity (also known as the "fight-flight-freeze" response), mediated by the release of epinephrine into the bloodstream. Signs of sympathetic arousal include elevated heart rate, rapid breathing, sweating, muscle tension, and dry mouth. We think of the sympathetic nervous system as functioning like an alarm system, which has become hypersensitive in individuals with anxiety-related disorders and must therefore be recalibrated. We will discuss how we incorporate this information into psychoeducation in chapter 2.

## Anxiety and Cognition

Cognitively, fearful responding can be characterized as maladaptive cognitive content (what the person thinks) and maladaptive cognitive process (how the person processes information). In terms of cognitive content, individuals with anxiety-related disorders are thought to be prone to *cognitive distortions* (A. T. Beck, Emery, & Greenberg, 1985), such as *probability overestimation* (magnifying the likelihood of a low-probability event) and *catastrophizing* (magnifying the impact or significance of a negative outcome, or "making a mountain out of a molehill"). For example:

- An individual with a fear of dogs might assume that dogs, even friendly ones, are going to bite him (*probability overestimation*).

- A client with social anxiety disorder might believe that if others see him sweat, he will be humiliated and will never recover (*catastrophizing*).

In terms of cognitive process, anxiety-related disorders are associated with an *attentional bias* toward threat-related cues (MacLeod, Mathews, & Tata, 1986): individuals with anxiety-related disorders chronically, and involuntarily, scan the environment for threat. For example:

- An individual with social anxiety giving a speech might disproportionately focus on the least-receptive members of the audience while ignoring audience members who appear more pleased and engaged in the speech.

- A client with PTSD related to interpersonal violence may constantly scan the environment, looking for "threatening" people.

- An individual with panic disorder may be hyper-attentive to any signs of physiological arousal, such as increased heart rate or lightheadedness.

## Anxiety and Behavior

Behaviorally, anxiety-related disorders are characterized by various forms of *avoidance*, and it is here that exposure therapy has its most direct impact. Some avoidance is of *external* stimuli (activities, situations, objects, or people that are external to the client). For example:

- An individual with agoraphobia might avoid driving or going to a crowded shopping mall.

- A person with contamination-related OCD might avoid coming into contact with things that appear dirty.

- A client with a specific phobia might avoid being near dogs, going to high places, or flying.

- A client with social anxiety might avoid speaking in public or interacting with others.

- An individual with motor vehicle accident-related PTSD might avoid driving on the highway.

- A child with separation anxiety disorder might avoid situations that involve being separated from caregivers, such as attending school.

- A client with illness anxiety disorder might avoid visiting the doctor for fear of getting bad news.

Avoidance can also be of *internal* stimuli, such as thoughts, emotions, or bodily sensations. For example:

- A person with panic disorder might go to great lengths to avoid experiencing elevated heart rate or dizziness by limiting exertion, caffeine intake, or emotional arousal.

- A client with PTSD might try to avoid memories of traumatic events.

- An individual with OCD might try to avoid "forbidden" or repugnant obsessive thoughts.

Other forms of avoidance (which can be obvious or not so obvious) involve *safety behaviors:* behaviors that the person feels will prevent a negative outcome or will reduce feelings of anxiety. For example:

- If a client with OCD accidentally touches something "dirty," he might wash his hands repeatedly or mentally reassure himself.

- A person with social anxiety disorder might interact with others at a party, but only after having a couple of drinks first.

- An individual with agoraphobia might go to the shopping mall, but only in the presence of a trusted companion.

- A client with motor vehicle accident-related PTSD may drive on the highway, but only in the right lane, at a slow speed, in light traffic.

## THE PROBLEM WITH AVOIDANCE

The impact of avoidance on fear is illustrated by a classic psychological experiment by Solomon, Kamin, and Wynne (1953). In this study, the researchers conditioned dogs to fear a light by shocking them at the same time that the light was turned on—a process called *fear conditioning*. They then turned their attention to the process of *fear extinction*: how the dogs "got over" the fear once it was learned. Fearful dogs were shown the "scary" light again and again, this time with no shock. Presumably, when dogs viewed the light over and over again, without being shocked, their fear would decrease. However, Solomon et al. added a twist: one group of dogs was allowed to escape the situation by jumping over a short wall; another group of dogs was not able to escape the situation. Results indicated that the dogs who could escape the situation—those who could jump over the wall and get away from the "scary" light—remained fearful indefinitely. Conversely, those dogs who had to remain in the situation were able to overcome the fear.

What does this tell us about anxiety-related disorders in humans? It tells us that avoidance tends to maintain fearful responding. The more we avoid, the more our fear persists and may even worsen. On the other hand, cessation of avoidance—*exposure*—leads to significant reductions in fear. Now, obviously, human clients are not identical to dogs in an experiment. We can't (and shouldn't) force our clients to face their fears, or physically prevent them from avoiding. But we can use our powers of persuasion to accomplish a similar effect. We need to help our clients understand that avoidance is part of the problem, and that exposure is the solution. In chapter 2, we will describe how you can use *psychoeducation* and *motivational interviewing* to help clients arrive at that conclusion.

## WHY DO EXPOSURE THERAPY?

By encouraging clients to face their fears, we are undermining the pattern of avoidant behavior and fearful responding. Exposure is thought to result in *inhibitory learning,* in which the brain adjusts to new information by showing that feared consequences are unlikely to occur and that distress is tolerable. We will discuss inhibitory learning in greater depth in chapter 3. From a cognitive perspective, exposure therapy helps combat the probability overestimation and catastrophizing associated with anxiety-related disorders. For example:

- An individual with panic disorder learns that he can experience an elevated heart rate without having a heart attack.

- The client with OCD learns that he does not become sick by touching "dirty" things.

- A socially anxious individual learns that minor blunders do not lead to his being ridiculed.

- The client with PTSD learns that he can remember the trauma without falling apart.

Ultimately, of course, the best argument for conducting exposure therapy comes from the clinical outcome data. Many well-conducted randomized controlled trials attest to the efficacy of exposure-based therapy for anxiety-related disorders. Meta-analysis, in which results from multiple studies are combined, demonstrates that exposure therapy is efficacious across the anxiety-related disorders (Hofmann & Smits, 2008; Norton & Price, 2007). Here are just a few examples from seminal research studies (italicized terms will be discussed in greater detail in subsequent chapters):

- A series of clients with specific phobias received one long session of *in vivo exposure*. At follow-up assessment (which ranged from 6 months to 7.5 years later; average 4 years), 65% of clients were described as having completely recovered. Another 25% were not recovered but were considered much improved (Öst, 1989).

- Individuals with social phobia were randomly assigned to receive a group CBT incorporating *in vivo exposure*, phenelzine, or placebo. Here we will focus on the efficacy of the exposure therapy. After twelve weeks of treatment, 75% of CBT treatment completers, versus 41% of placebo treatment completers, were considered treatment responders. Exposure therapy and phenelzine had equivalent response rates (Heimberg et al., 1998).

- Individuals with panic disorder were randomized to receive a CBT that prioritized *interoceptive exposure* and *in vivo exposure*, imipramine, combination treatment, or placebo. Immediately after treatment, 49% of exposure recipients, compared to 22% of placebo recipients, were considered treatment responders. Six months after treatment discontinuation, 32% of exposure recipients, versus 13% of placebo recipients, were considered treatment responders. Exposure therapy and imipramine had equivalent short-term effects, with some potential advantage for combined treatment; however, after treatment was discontinued, clients who received exposure therapy (with or without imipramine) showed a lower rate of relapse (Barlow, Gorman, Shear, & Woods, 2000).

- Clients with OCD were assigned to receive *exposure with response prevention*, clomipramine, combination treatment, or placebo. After twelve weeks of treatment, 86% of those who completed exposure treatment, compared to 10% of placebo recipients, were considered responders. Exposure therapy was superior to clomipramine (Foa et al., 2005).

These results appear to hold up in "real-world" clinical settings as well as in academic research settings. In fact, across studies, exposure-based treatments conducted in nonacademic clinics and hospitals, with clinically representative clients, seem to be about as effective as they are in more carefully controlled, laboratory-based trials (Hans & Hiller, 2013; Stewart & Chambless, 2009).

## The Perils of Exposophobia

Schare and Wyatt (2013) used the tongue-in-cheek term *exposophobia* to refer to "the extreme fear (and associated avoidance) of using exposure therapy procedures occurring in trained mental health professionals" (p. 252). Indeed, exposure therapy is grossly underused by mental health therapists (e.g., Becker, Zayfert, & Anderson, 2004; Goisman et al., 1993). Given the solid theoretical and empirical background for the use of exposure therapy in anxiety-related disorders, what might account for this underutilization? In many cases, it appears that therapists fear upsetting the client or damaging the therapeutic relationship. This is due, in part, to several myths about exposure (see Tolin, 2016), described below.

### *Exposophobia Myth 1: Exposure will cause intolerable anxiety.*

It is true that exposure, by design, produces temporary feelings of anxiety. However, the available evidence shows that this increased anxiety is neither long-lasting nor intolerable, so long as the exposure is conducted thoughtfully and in collaboration with the client. In one study of clients with PTSD, approximately one-quarter reported a temporary increase in feelings of anxiety in the days following exposure. Those who reported an exacerbation of anxiety benefited just as much from the treatment in the long run as did those whose anxiety did not increase (Foa, Zoellner, Feeny, Hembree, & Alvarez-Conrad, 2002).

### *Exposophobia Myth 2: Exposure will increase co-occurring problems, such as substance abuse.*

Exposure therapy has been examined in clients with co-occurring PTSD and substance use disorders. These studies show that the clients reported *reductions* in substance use, as well as reductions in their PTSD symptoms (Berenz, Rowe, Schumacher, Stasiewicz, & Coffey, 2012; Brady, Dansky, Back, Foa, & Carroll, 2001; Mills et al., 2012). We might opt to have dually diagnosed clients receive specialized substance abuse treatment concurrently with exposure therapy, but the evidence doesn't suggest that we should avoid using exposure with such clients.

### *Exposophobia Myth 3: Exposure should not be used for PTSD, childhood sexual abuse, or complex PTSD.*

A wealth of empirical evidence shows that exposure therapy is effective in a wide range of clients with PTSD, including motor vehicle accident survivors, combat veterans, rape victims, and survivors of childhood sexual trauma (Powers, Halpern, Ferenschak,

Gillihan, & Foa, 2010). Indeed, exposure-based therapy has been identified as the only psychological intervention with high strength of evidence for PTSD (Institute of Medicine, 2008; Jonas et al., 2013), and it is considered a first-line treatment for clients with complex PTSD (Cloitre et al., 2011). We'll discuss exposure therapy for PTSD in greater detail in chapter 9.

### Exposophobia Myth 4: Exposure with children should be avoided.

Several studies demonstrate that children actually respond quite well to exposure-based therapy (see Kendall et al., 2006). The efficacy of exposure therapy in children has been demonstrated in children as young as preschool age (Lewin et al., 2014). Other studies with children and adolescents show that exposure is effective in the treatment of pediatric phobias (Ollendick et al., 2009), panic disorder (Pincus, May, Whitton, Mattis, & Barlow, 2010), OCD (Franklin et al., 2015), and PTSD (Gilboa-Schechtman et al., 2010). In chapter 4, we will talk more about specific applications of exposure therapy with children.

### Exposophobia Myth 5: Clients don't want or can't tolerate exposure therapy.

Contrary to this myth, the evidence shows that clients find exposure acceptable. When student trauma survivors and women with PTSD were given a choice between exposure therapy and antidepressant medications, they were three to four times more likely to choose exposure therapy than they were to choose medication (Becker, Darius, & Schaumberg, 2007; Zoellner, Feeny, Cochran, & Pruitt, 2003). Furthermore, exposure is not associated with increased dropout rates. Across studies of PTSD, clients are no more likely to drop out of exposure therapy than they are to drop out of other psychological treatments (Hembree et al., 2003). In studies where clients were assigned to receive exposure vs. pharmacotherapy, dropout rates were generally equivalent (Barlow et al., 2000; Foa et al., 2005; Heimberg et al., 1998).

### Exposophobia Myth 6: Exposure therapy must be prefaced by extensive coping skill training.

In our clinical experience, we find that many, if not most, clients do not require coping skill training and can dive into exposure therapy right away. However, some clients do require significant coping skill training, though this is more of the exception rather than a rule. As one example, dialectical behavioral therapy (a CBT variant specifically designed for clients with borderline personality disorder and/or repeated self-injurious behavior) employs exposure for PTSD symptoms but prefaces this exposure with emotion regulation skill training (Linehan, 2014). Some studies of PTSD suggest that coping skill training prior to exposure therapy may decrease dropout rates and improve efficacy (Bryant et al., 2013; Cloitre et al., 2010).

## Going Beyond "Normal"

A common misconception of exposure therapy is that it is designed to mimic "normal" human behavior. Certainly, some of the things our clients avoid, and to which we want to expose them, are the kinds of things that people without anxiety disorders do every day. In exposure therapy, we might ask our clients to perform "normal" behaviors, such as:

- Driving

- Eating in a restaurant

- Talking to people

- Going to school or work

- Shopping in a mall

But we might also ask our clients to do some decidedly "abnormal" things, such as:

- Hyperventilating

- Listening to audio recordings of stories of traumatic experiences

- Touching a toilet with bare hands

- Talking to people after dabbing water on one's forehead to simulate sweat

Why go to such lengths with exposure? Why not just prescribe "normal" behavior? One reason is that it is difficult to predict what clients will encounter in real life, and we want to make sure that our clients are adequately prepared for whatever experiences they might have, even unanticipated ones. In addition, if you "overshoot" some of the exposures by doing things that are more challenging than the client is likely to have to face in everyday life, then the everyday tasks and roadblocks later on won't seem so bad. This is because the client will already have mastered much more challenging and higher-level exposures. For example, if a client with OCD agrees to an exposure in which he touches a toilet with his bare hands and then touches his face, hair, and clothes without washing afterward, imagine how much easier it will be for him when he needs to ride the subway to work, shake hands with someone, or use public bathrooms.

Second, and perhaps more critical, is the fact that low-grade exposures teach a message of *conditional safety* (Otto, Simon, Olatunji, Sung, & Pollack, 2011): "I'm safe *if...*" For example, a client with social anxiety might interact with others and learn the conditional safety lesson "I'm safe *if* others don't see me sweating." A client with OCD might use a public bathroom and learn the conditional safety lesson "I'm safe *if* my hands don't touch the toilet." A client with panic disorder might go to the mall and learn the conditional safety lesson "I'm safe *if* I keep my breathing under control and stay relaxed." We want the client to learn a lesson of *unconditional safety:* "I'm safe, period."

## A Note About Risk

After reading the last section, you might be wondering where we draw the line when it comes to safety. Certainly, we do not want to create unnecessary risk of harm for our clients. But we also don't want to do subtherapeutic treatment. We find it helpful to talk through these issues with our clients and to help them recognize that 100 percent safety is an irrational goal. Part of living a happy life is being willing to tolerate certain risks.

Perhaps it's helpful to think about all of the risks that are present, but that we don't even think of, during our day-to-day experience. Let's imagine a typical client's day. He wakes up and, like many people with anxiety-related disorders, takes his antidepressant or benzodiazepine medication. Then he gets in the car and drives on city streets or on a highway to get to your office. He then has a session of exposure therapy with you. Which is the most dangerous of these activities? Which is the least dangerous? It's worth considering the fact that we routinely advise clients to take medications, despite the fact that these medications can have significant adverse effects. And we routinely ask our clients to drive to our office, despite the fact that motor vehicle accidents are a leading cause of death. Now, to be clear, we are not anti-medication, nor are we anti-driving. We raise these issues to make the point that life has risks, and we decide that certain risks are worth taking. So it is with exposure therapy. Our aim in planning exposures is therefore not to determine whether a given activity is 100 percent safe, but rather to determine whether it is safe *enough*.

# CONCLUSIONS

Many people will experience an anxiety-related disorder in their lifetime. This is often accompanied by financial, social, and work-related distress. Fortunately, exposure therapy is an empirically supported treatment that is used to help treat the anxiety, phobia, panic, PTSD, or other disorder. Some clinicians have had misconceptions about using exposure with clients (e.g., it could worsen anxiety, children aren't able to handle it, or it is unsafe to do unless clients are equipped with extensive coping skills). However, we have outlined why it is safe and effective to use this in your work with clients, and why it is important to combat exposophobia.

The next chapter will be dedicated to pitching the idea of exposure therapy to your client. One of the most important components of this "pitch" is to have confidence in the treatment as well as in your delivery of the treatment. We will highlight the importance of providing psychoeducation to clients and working collaboratively with them. Some clients may be ambivalent about making a change in their lives, so we will also discuss principles of motivational interviewing.

# CHAPTER 2

# Getting Clients on Board

Fundamentally, exposure therapy is about getting clients to do things that they would rather avoid. That aim often requires a good deal of persuasion—in essence, "pitching" the concept of exposure to a sometimes-skeptical client. CBT is a combination of art and science, and there is definitely an art to the pitch. The pitch is important not only because we want the client to choose exposure therapy, but also because we want the client to feel confident in the treatment and comfortable with you as a therapist.

There are many different components to a good exposure pitch. These include:

- Providing your client with psychoeducation about her disorder, the model of treatment, and the likelihood for success

- Establishing therapeutic rapport

- Using motivational interviewing strategies to assess the client's stage of change

- Developing a collaborative working relationship

- Modeling exposures for the client

In this chapter, we'll walk you through each of these steps.

## USING PSYCHOEDUCATION

Psychoeducation doesn't mean lecturing the client. Rather, psychoeducation involves a back-and-forth conversation in which the therapist asks questions and provides information to help the client understand the topic. Good psychoeducation regarding exposure therapy involves providing the client with a model of anxiety and explaining how avoidance is the enemy.

### Providing a Model of Anxiety

CBT is based on the notion that fear (or any other emotion) can be conceptualized as a triangle of thoughts, feelings, and behaviors (see figure 1). Fearful *thoughts* include the probability overestimation and catastrophizing we mentioned in chapter 1. Clients tend to believe that bad outcomes are highly likely, and they tend to believe that such bad outcomes will be not merely bad; they will be disastrous, or catastrophic. Fearful *feelings* include the subjective emotional state of fear, along with the accompanying "fight-flight-freeze" physiological reactions such as elevated heart rate, rapid breathing, sweating, muscle tension, and dry mouth. Fearful *behaviors* include avoidance as well as safety behaviors. The bidirectional arrows in figure 1 indicate that an increase in one component tends to lead to increases in the other components. As people think more fearfully, they tend to feel and behave more fearfully as well. As people feel more fearful, they tend to think and act more fearfully. And as people behave more fearfully, their fearful thoughts and feelings are maintained, thus creating a vicious cycle.

One of our first tasks is to help the client understand this triangle of thoughts, feelings, and behaviors, which we refer to as the CBT triangle. Here's an example of starting the psychoeducation discussion with a client.

*Therapist:*    I'm going to introduce what our treatment is going to look like, and I will give you a chance to ask me any questions you may have. First, we need to understand that all of our thoughts, feelings, and behaviors are linked together. That is, this problem that you're experiencing has something to do with how you think, and something to do with how you feel, and something to do with how you act. Does that make sense?

*Client:*    I'm not sure. Can you explain what you mean?

*Therapist:*    Here, let me draw this on a piece of paper (draws the diagram shown in figure 1). You see here I have your thoughts, your feelings, and your behaviors all interconnecting. That's what the problem looks like, if we break it down. But let's take it one piece at a time. The "thoughts" part refers to the thoughts you have when something upsets you. These are the words or ideas that go through your head. Can you think of some thoughts that you've had when something bothered you?

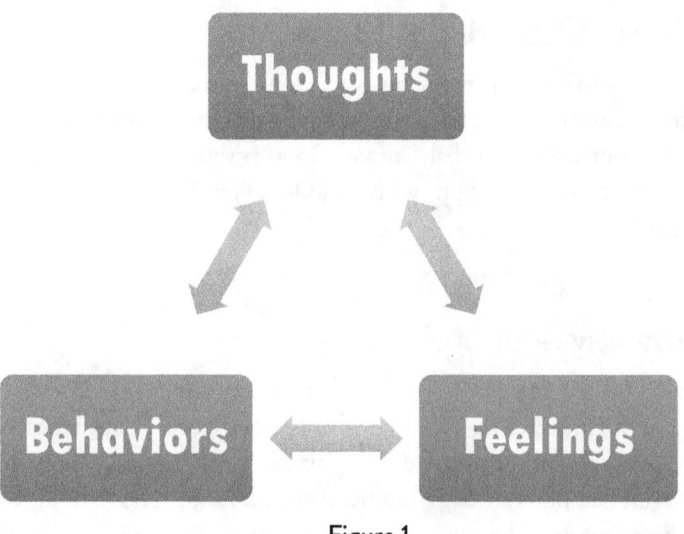

Figure 1

*Client:*  Yeah, I guess when I see something dirty, I think the germs are going to get on me and make me sick. Is that what you mean?

*Therapist:* Yes, that's exactly what I mean. How we think about things often plays a big role in how we feel about them. For example, when you think that germs are going to get on you, and you're going to get sick, how do you feel then?

*Client:*  I feel nervous and anxious.

*Therapist:* Okay, nervous and anxious. Those are feelings, and it's very understandable that you'd feel that way, if you're thinking something's going to make you sick. I suspect a lot of people would feel anxious if they thought they were going to get sick. And how we think and feel is closely linked to what we do. So let's come back to your example. Here you are, thinking that germs are going to get on you, and you're going to get sick. What do you do?

*Client:*  Well, the main thing is that I don't touch the thing that looks dirty.

*Therapist:* Exactly. So part of the behavior here is what you don't do. You don't touch things that look dirty. We call that "avoidance." And if you do feel like some germs might be on you, what do you do then?

*Client:*  I have to wash my hands over and over until they feel clean again.

*Therapist:* Yes, so another part of your behavior is what you do do. You wash your hands. We call that a "safety behavior." Can you imagine why we call it that?

*Client:*  Because it makes me feel safer?

*Therapist:* Yes, that's it exactly. So you see that your thoughts, your feelings, and your behaviors are all linked—and the therapy I have in mind for you is designed to help all three of those components.

## Making Avoidance the Enemy

Exposure therapy is designed to counteract the vicious cycle of avoidance and fear. Remember, avoidance can be of external factors (e.g., certain situations, objects, or people), or it can be of internal factors (e.g., certain thoughts, memories, or bodily sensations). Regardless of what is being avoided, the net result is the same—it is perceived as more threatening over time, and the person is deprived of the opportunity to challenge the fear and eventually overcome it. Therefore, in our psychoeducation, we take time to help the client understand the toxic role of avoidance in maintaining the problem.

*Therapist:* I want to talk about avoidant behaviors a little more. You've mentioned that you have some things that you don't do, like not touching things that seem dirty, and some things that you do do, like washing your hands. What, do you suppose, is the effect of those behaviors on your fear?

*Client:*       Well, I know when I wash my hands I feel better. And it feels better not to touch things that are dirty.

*Therapist:*    Yes, so there's a short-term relief from avoidance and safety behaviors, right? You wash your hands and you feel better; you avoid and you feel better. How about in the long term? What do you think is the long-term effect on you?

*Client:*       I'm not sure I understand.

*Therapist:*    Well, imagine it this way. Let's say I am deathly afraid of, I don't know, tuna fish sandwiches. And I come to you as my therapist for help. Can you imagine that?

*Client:*       (laughs) Okay.

*Therapist:*    And let's say I'm really bothered by this fear. It's really messing up my life because I can't go to anyone's house where there might be a tuna fish sandwich, I can't go to restaurants, and so on. With me so far?

*Client:*       Yeah.

*Therapist:*    So I tell you, my way of coping with this fear is to make sure I never go near a tuna fish sandwich. Not only will I not go near them, I won't look at them, I won't go anywhere there might be one, I won't even say the word "tuna." And if I do accidentally see a tuna fish sandwich, I go home and take a shower. All of these actions—this avoidance and these safety behaviors—make me feel a little better. In the long run, what's likely to happen to my fear of tuna fish sandwiches?

*Client:*       Well, I don't think it's going to go away.

*Therapist:*    I don't think so either. Why not?

*Client:*       Well, because if you always avoid tuna fish sandwiches, then you'll never get to see that they're okay and can't hurt you.

*Therapist:*    That's exactly right. I never give myself a chance to learn anything different. So my avoidance and my safety behaviors make me feel a little better in the short term, but in the long term they actually hurt me and can even make my fear of tuna fish sandwiches worse. Now let's talk about your situation and use that same logic. Your avoidance and your safety behaviors make you feel a little better in the short term, right? What, do you suppose, is the long-term effect on you?

*Client:*       They keep me afraid?

*Therapist:* Exactly right. They keep you stuck where you are. As long as you're doing these safety behaviors and this avoidance, you're going to keep being afraid. Now, as my therapist, what would you recommend for my tuna fish fear? Should I keep avoiding and doing my safety behaviors?

*Client:* No, you should probably eat a tuna fish sandwich so you can get over it.

*Therapist:* I like where you're going with this, but what if that's just too scary for me right now?

*Client:* Well, I suppose you could start small, like maybe just saying "tuna" or something like that.

*Therapist:* Ah, taking a gradual approach. I like that. What then?

*Client:* And then you could, for example, look at pictures of tuna fish sandwiches, and then be around tuna fish sandwiches in real life, and eventually work your way up to eating one.

*Therapist:* Yes, we can take it step by step until the goal is reached. And this is exactly what we will be doing together to help you overcome your fears.

## Explaining How Exposure Works

As you can see in the above example, the therapist has used a nonfrightening metaphor to segue into a discussion of graded exposure. Here, the therapist talks in more detail about how the therapy will work.

*Therapist:* Let's go back to this diagram of thoughts, feelings, and behaviors. A big goal of our therapy is to break down the interactions among these three parts. One of the main ways we will do this is through a strategy called exposure, which targets the "behaviors" part of the triangle. Specifically, our job is to identify those times where you're likely to engage in avoidance or use a safety behavior, and do the opposite—to approach, rather than avoid. The "thoughts" component of the triangle is also important. I may ask you to challenge some of the ways you think about things, or to test things out to see if your way of thinking is accurate—to be on the lookout for evidence that either confirms or contradicts some of the thoughts that you have. Many times the evidence that we gather to challenge your thoughts will come directly from the exposures that we do together. For example, if you are afraid of touching contaminated items, like pens or door handles, since you fear you could get sick, we may touch the things you are afraid of again and again and again until your body and your brain learn that nothing bad happens. Therefore, the exposure will likely change the way you think about those contaminated items.

*Client:*      But why do it again and again? Can't we just do the exposure once and be done with it?

*Therapist:*    I wouldn't recommend doing that, and here's why: if you complete an exposure where you touch a door handle one time and you don't get sick, your brain may later think that nothing bad happened because that particular door handle was okay and just happened to be "safe." So, in a way, the exposure that you may have worked so hard on in the session was discounted. But, let's say you touched 100 different door handles in the course of exposure therapy. Then it would be pretty hard for your brain to discount them all and say all of those exposures were "lucky" in that they weren't contaminated or didn't get you sick.

*Client:*      That makes sense.

## Having a Conversation About Fear

It is important to have a discussion with your client about the nature of fear. For example, you might ask your client, "Do you think fear is harmful or dangerous?" Some clients will know that it really isn't dangerous, whereas others are convinced that fear or physical arousal must be avoided at all costs. Some clients, particularly (though not limited to) those with panic disorder or agoraphobia, may say that they fear the long-term consequences of fear and think it could lead to a heart attack, accident, "going crazy," or other aversive outcome. This is why a discussion of the nature of fear is critical, as it establishes an important piece of the foundation for your work together.

Fear is uncomfortable, but not dangerous. In fact, under the right circumstances, fear can be quite adaptive. Here, the therapist uses psychoeducation to help the client distinguish between adaptive and maladaptive fear.

*Therapist:*    Obviously we've been talking about how your fear has caused problems for you. But I also want to point out that fear, by itself, is not a bad emotion. It's actually helpful and necessary. Can you imagine what it would be like if a person had zero fear—couldn't even feel it?

*Client:*      It sounds great, to be honest. I wish I had zero fear.

*Therapist:*    It might seem great, but imagine what would happen if a person with zero fear stepped into traffic and there was a car heading toward him?

*Client:*      I guess he wouldn't get out of the way and he'd get run over.

*Therapist:*    Right. It's fear, in measured doses, that gets you to jump back up onto the sidewalk when you see a car coming. Some amount of fear is really important. It keeps us on our toes and often protects us from harm. I really want to emphasize that: fear is not inherently bad. The problem is that for some people, the fear turns on when it doesn't need to. It doesn't wait for an oncoming car, for example. It just turns on even when nothing dangerous is happening. Let's call that a "false alarm." Your brain and body are having a fear reaction even when there's no danger. Part of our work during exposure therapy will involve understanding when these false alarms are sounding, and how to handle them differently from how you have handled them in the past, such as through avoidance and safety behaviors.

You can have a discussion with your client about the various physiological symptoms of anxiety and how they were designed to protect you. This list, adapted from Craske and Barlow (2006), is a helpful guide:

- Increased heart and respiration rate functions to get more oxygenated blood to the muscles associated with running.

- Tingling in the extremities or face (paresthesias) is a result of blood being redirected toward the big muscle groups associated with flight.

- Sweating cools the body and makes it slippery (harder to catch).

- Dry mouth and stomach discomfort are the result of a partial shutdown of the digestive system to free up energy for muscles, which will help the person fight or flee.

- Lightheadedness and dizziness are often byproducts of hyperventilation, taking more air into the body (which would be adaptive if the person were actually running or fighting).

You may also talk with your client about the natural course of anxiety. What goes up must eventually come down, meaning that anxiety can't stay elevated forever. The body is designed to protect you. Therefore, the anxiety will eventually lower on its own without the client doing anything to make it come down.

## Emphasizing Exposure's Effectiveness

While you should be careful not to overpromise results, it's important to point out that this treatment really does work (as discussed in very abbreviated form in chapter 1). Of course, success in treatment depends on many different factors. It depends on the extent to which your clients do what you encourage them to do in session, as well as the extent to which they complete homework assignments outside of the session. It also depends on clients' motivation level, level of confidence in the treatment, and other factors that we, as therapists, can influence, such as our level of confidence in our clients (which can greatly impact the confidence they have about themselves in the treatment), how well we listen to our clients, and how well we work as a team to treat the disorder. Here's a script illustrating how to discuss the effectiveness of treatment with your client.

*Therapist:*     Let's talk a little bit about the effectiveness of exposure therapy. I wonder whether any questions have come up for you about that.

*Client:*      Yeah, I was wondering how likely this is to be successful for me.

*Therapist:*   The bottom line is that it's highly likely to be successful for you. But I want to clarify what I mean by "successful," because it's important that we have a realistic understanding of what to expect. "Success," in my view, doesn't mean that you'll never feel fear again. As we discussed, fear is a very normal human emotion, and it will be part of your life, just like it's part of everyone else's life, forever. But what we can reasonably expect is that we can get this fear "out of your face." We can get it to the point where it's no longer troubling you day in and day out, that it no longer has control of your actions, and that it no longer impairs your ability to do things you want to do. Does that make sense?

*Client:*      Yes. Will the results be permanent?

*Therapist:*   Here's what the scientific evidence tells us. First, when people have a good response to exposure therapy, as I think you will, more often than not they tend to continue showing a good response at long-term follow-up assessments. That's the good news. On the other hand, it's also important to understand what's happening in exposure therapy at a very basic level. Exposure doesn't "erase" your fear or zap it out of your brain. It's still in there. Rather, through the course of exposure, you learn something new—like how to cope by approaching, rather than avoiding—and that new habit becomes stronger over time. But there is always a possibility that an old fear habit can come back over time, in response to stress, or under new conditions. Fortunately, our experience has been that if and when the fear pops back up, you can get back on the program and get it back under control.

# ESTABLISHING RAPPORT

No matter what your theoretical orientation is as a therapist, you know that rapport is one of the most critical aspects of treatment. We want our clients to know that we seek to understand what they are going through, appreciate their willingness to come to therapy and try something new, and are confident that we can help them feel better.

Let your clients know that you want their feedback about treatment and about the therapeutic relationship. This also shows your clients that you are interested in their thoughts about how treatment is going and are willing to make corrective steps, if needed. Be ready to be flexible and modify your treatment. If the rapport becomes ruptured in any way, you should work to repair the rupture by directly addressing what happened, taking nondefensive ownership for your role in the rupture, and asking for client feedback (for additional discussion see Safran, Muran, & Eubanks-Carter, 2011).

# USING MOTIVATIONAL INTERVIEWING

A full discussion of *motivational interviewing* (MI) is outside the scope of this book; interested readers are directed to Miller and Rollnick (2013). MI is based on the idea that motivation to change behaviors, engage in treatment, and take other actions can fluctuate over time. At any given time, a client's *stage of change* (Prochaska & DiClemente, 1982)—her awareness of the problem, readiness to work on it, and willingness to stick with a treatment plan—could be defined as (a) *precontemplation* (not acknowledging the problem or not being willing to change), (b) *contemplation* ("waffling," being unsure about whether or not to change the behavior), (c) *action* (deciding to work on the problem and beginning the process of changing), or (d) *maintenance* (continuing to work on the problem and trying to prevent backsliding).

A good way to think about MI is that our job, as therapists, is to escort the client from one stage of change to the next. That is, if the client is in the precontemplation stage, our job is to escort her to the contemplation stage; if the client is the contemplation stage, our job is to escort her to the action stage; and if the client is in the action stage, our job is to escort her to the maintenance stage.

## Escorting the Client from Precontemplation to Contemplation

The precontemplative client is stuck, and our job is to get her unstuck. We want to get the discussion started, avoid argumentative pitfalls, and get the client considering alternatives. Here are some helpful strategies:

**Avoid argumentation.** At this stage, resist the urge to try to convince the client that she has a problem, or that she needs to do exposure therapy. Such efforts are likely to just trigger counterarguments. Instead, simply get the client talking about the issue.

**Roll with resistance.** When the client says something like "I don't think I need therapy," don't try to persuade her otherwise. Trying to persuade a precontemplative client doesn't seem to help, and it often backfires. Instead, try just reflecting back what she said so the client knows you've heard it.

**Develop discrepancy.** Talk to you client about her larger goals and values—not just as they relate to the presenting problem. What does your client want her life to look like? What is truly important to her? Reflect this back to the client and ask her to compare and contrast these goals and values with her current behavior, which might sound like this: "It sounds like you're in a tough spot right now. On one hand, you're not sure you like the idea of being in therapy, and you really don't like the idea of being labeled as having an 'anxiety problem.' On the other hand, your work is very important to you, but you're noticing that lately you have been avoiding talking to your colleagues and supervisor because of anxious feelings. I wonder how you reconcile that."

## Escorting the Client from Contemplation to Action

The client in the contemplation stage is waffling. She is entertaining the idea that there is a problem and/or that she needs help. Our job is to help this client decide what to do. Here are the major strategies:

**Weigh pros and cons.** Get out a piece of paper and draw a line down the middle. Label one side "pros," and the other "cons." Ask the client questions such as "What would be some of the benefits or positives of doing this treatment?" "What would be some of the costs or negatives?" "What would be the pros and cons of just leaving things where they are?" "Which strategy is most likely to help you reach your goals in life?"

**Invite change talk.** The philosopher Pascal (1623–1662) wrote, "People are better persuaded by the reasons they themselves discovered than those that come into the minds of others." That is, the client, not the therapist, should make the argument for changing. You can influence this by asking key questions such as "What makes you think this is a problem?" or "What steps do you think you need to take in order to feel better?"

**Avoid uninvited prescriptions.** The client in the contemplation stage may not be ready to accept your opinion that she needs treatment, and that suggestion on your part may just trigger a counterargument and send the client back to the precontemplation stage. Offer an opinion only if asked, and if so, do it gently and try to provide more than one option (e.g., CBT, medication management, self-help books).

## Escorting the Client from Action to Maintenance

The client in the action stage has made up her mind to start treatment. We now want to get her actively working on the problem, which we do using the following two strategies:

**Make a plan.** Work collaboratively with your client to develop the treatment plan, including how many sessions you'll have (at least a rough idea), how often you'll meet, what kinds of exposures you'll do, and expectations for homework (yes, there will be homework!). Make sure that the client feels like an active partner in this process.

**Periodically reassess stage of change.** Don't overestimate the client's motivation. Stages of change can be slippery, and it's easy for a client in the action stage, for example, to slide back into contemplation instead of forward into maintenance. Therefore, watch for emerging signs of resistance and check in with the client about her stage of change as needed.

# COLLABORATING AS CO-SCIENTISTS

As the old saying goes, two heads are better than one, and this is certainly the case in exposure therapy. *Collaborative empiricism* is a core aspect of CBT and enhances the therapeutic relationship. Think of your client as your co-scientist, and be on the hunt together to form and test hypotheses through exposure. Share with your client at the first session that she will have a very active role in treatment. Your discussion with the client may go something like this:

> *The two of us are going to work together in this treatment. While my expertise is in treating anxiety disorders, you know your own anxiety much better than I ever will. You know the ins and outs of it, what makes it worse, and what things you have been doing to try to feel better. Therefore, I'll ask you to share with me what is working and what isn't. This treatment is a team effort. I find the therapy is much more effective, and easier to stick with, when we come up with ideas together and give each other feedback.*

Working together in this fashion not only builds rapport, but also allows the client to learn how to be thinking and what to be doing outside of the session. One of the goals of therapy is getting the client to feel well informed and confident enough to design and implement her own exposures once the therapy has ended.

# MODELING

It is preferable to do exposure *with* your clients, if at all possible. This can show them that you are willing to take risks as well. For example, if you are asking a client with OCD to walk into the bathroom with you and touch a germy toilet, then you had best be ready to touch that toilet yourself! However, if it is clear that the client will have a much easier time doing the exposure with you (perhaps because you are serving as a *safety signal*, a sign that the exposure is safe), then you may want to consider having her do the exposure by herself. For example, let's say that your client has a fear of enclosed spaces and is about to ride an elevator. You might opt to accompany the client into the elevator and ride with her for a couple of sessions. However, it is possible that your presence becomes a safety signal for the client (e.g., *I know I'm going to be okay because my therapist is here and can perform CPR if I have a heart attack* or *My therapist will know just what to do if this elevator gets stuck*). In such a case, subsequent exposures should be conducted without your presence.

## CONCLUSIONS

In this chapter, we have discussed specific ways to get the client's buy-in for exposure therapy. This treatment is all about reversing old patterns of avoidant behavior, so perhaps it's not surprising that some clients require a bit of "selling." The biggest element of our pitch is psychoeducational. Most clients, once they understand the model of anxiety and the relationships among thoughts, feelings, and behaviors—especially avoidant behaviors—will readily understand that exposure is the way to go. Still, some clients, quite understandably, are fearful about the prospect of replacing their avoidance with approach. The motivational interviewing strategies of avoiding argumentation, rolling with resistance, and developing discrepancy are quite helpful in persuading clients in the precontemplation stage of change that they might need to reconsider their stance. For contemplative clients, weighing pros and cons and inviting change talk while avoiding uninvited prescriptions can help them settle on exposure as a preferred treatment strategy. And for clients in the action stage, making a plan and not overestimating their motivation will help them maintain their initiative. Finally, once the client is on board with exposure, the strategies of collaborative empiricism and modeling will help keep the client engaged.

In the next chapter, we will provide the basic guidelines for exposure. We will not only give examples of the various types of exposures but will also describe how to best implement them in session with your client.

# CHAPTER 3

# General Parameters of Exposure

As we discussed in chapter 1, anxiety-related disorders are maintained, in part, by the client's avoidance of feared external and/or internal stimuli. In exposure therapy, our job is to help our clients to face their fears systematically by repeatedly confronting feared objects, activities, situations, thoughts, or feelings.

In this chapter, we will guide you through the various types of exposures and provide instruction for implementing each type. We will also discuss models of exposure, including the *habituation* model and the *inhibitory learning* model. When you read part 2 of this book, which consists of exposure ideas for many anxiety-related disorders, we encourage you to design and implement the exposures using the information included in this chapter in order to best help your client have a successful exposure session.

## TYPES OF EXPOSURE EXERCISES

There are four main types of exposures that can be used throughout therapy and that we'll discuss in this chapter:

- In vivo exposure

- Imaginal exposure

- Exposure to thoughts

- Exposure to body sensations (also known as interoceptive exposures)

In addition to the above-mentioned exposures, we address how to use virtual reality in therapy. Virtual reality is another way to target feared sensations and thoughts as well as allow the client to have a more immersive imaginal exposure experience.

### In Vivo Exposure

In vivo exposure is the type of exposure that most easily comes to mind when thinking about exposure therapy. This form of exposure consists of directly confronting feared situations in real life. In vivo exposures can be conducted with your client in or outside of the therapy office or can be assigned to your client for homework.

## Examples of In Vivo Exposure

In vivo exposure can take countless forms. Some examples include:

- A client with a snake phobia holds a snake.

- A client with fear of flying goes on an airplane.

- A client with a fear of giving a speech in front of an audience.

- A client with OCD touches things that seem dirty or germy.

When designing in vivo exposures, make sure that they are safe for the client (and you too!). We are not asking you to take your clients to dark alleys at night in big cities with money hanging out of their pockets to target their fears of getting mugged or attacked. Similarly, we are not asking you to take your client with a phobia of snakes into the wild to try to provoke a dangerous snake. We do, however, want you to design challenging exposures with your clients. For your client with fears of being mugged, walking through the city alone is likely a "safe enough" thing to do. For your client with a snake phobia who won't even go out into the garden for fear that a snake will be there, we want him to work in her garden as an exposure and to take appropriate risks.

## Guidelines for Setting up In Vivo Exposures

Sometimes with in vivo exposure, we ask clients to do things that are decidedly abnormal. For example, if your client is afraid of germs and you want to expose her to potential contaminants, you might ask her to touch trash dumpsters and then smear those germs all over her clothes, hair, and face. Most people don't do such things on an everyday basis—but, as we discussed in chapter 1, we usually have to go beyond "normal" behavior in order for your client to get better. So, yes, things can get a little odd. Here's an example of a conversation you could have with a client about what to expect when moving forward with exposure therapy.

| | |
|---|---|
| *Therapist:* | I know you said that one of your main concerns is that you will vomit. You've mentioned that you avoid talking about vomiting for fear that it will make you throw up, and that you stay away from people who have been sick because you're concerned that they could contaminate you and make you throw up. |
| *Client:* | Yeah, that's been my worst fear for a long time now. I've become really good at avoiding all sorts of places in which I could get sick. |
| *Therapist:* | I understand that has been really scary for you. Working together, we will soon be creating a list, or hierarchy, of exposures that we will work on together in session and that you will do outside of session for homework. For example, we might begin with exposures of looking at pictures of vomit or watching videos of people vomiting, and then move on to more challenging exposures such as going near people who are sick or pretending to throw up. |

*Client:*     I get that I will have to do some challenging things, but going near people who are sick on purpose is kind of weird. I don't know anyone else who has to do that in their everyday life.

*Therapist:*  That's a great point. It's important to recognize that some of the things we do will seem kind of weird, and they won't be what people typically do in their everyday lives. Your anxiety tells you an awful lot of scary lies about how bad things are and how sick you will get. The best way to fight back is to confront your fear of getting sick that your anxiety doesn't want you to confront, including the really hard stuff, like sitting in a hospital waiting room since there are likely to be people there who recently vomited. If we just decided to stop treatment after you watched some videos of people vomiting, then I bet it would be pretty darn scary if you were later around a friend who had recently had the flu or some other illness. If we can create challenging exposures now, then most things you will encounter naturally in the real world will seem insignificant compared to what you have already mastered.

*Client:*     That makes sense.

*Therapist:*  Great. I do want to point out that I will never force you to do anything that you don't want to do or don't feel ready to do. While I want each exposure to be a challenge, I also want you to succeed.

## Imaginal Exposure

When in vivo exposure is not possible or practical, such as with the client who fears plane crashes or who has had a traumatic experience (e.g., assault, natural disaster), you can use imaginal exposure. Imaginal exposure involves creating a narrative either on paper, on a computer, or on a mobile device that the client will read aloud (or listen to a recording of) repeatedly until the fear is reduced. In the narrative, you will want to the client to include vivid details and to include as much sensory information as possible (what the client sees, hears, and smells in the feared situation) to bring the fear into the present moment for a powerful exposure.

### Examples of Imaginal Exposure

The following are examples of imaginal exposure:

- A client with PTSD deliberately recalls the memory of a traumatic event in vivid detail.

- An individual with OCD writes a detailed story about dying of a terrible disease because he didn't wash his hands.

- A client with a fear of flying deliberately imagines being on a violently turbulent flight, records the story into his phone, and listens to it repeatedly.

Imaginal exposure doesn't have to be reserved for exposure items that can't be recreated in vivo. It can also be an important part of your client's hierarchy of fears earlier in treatment to help him gradually work up to doing in vivo exposure. For example, if your client has a fear of contamination, you might consider doing an imaginal exposure in which he writes a detailed story about becoming contaminated, how the contamination occurred, and the feared outcome, such as contracting a disease. This may be a stepping-stone toward later doing in vivo exposure in which you ask your client to touch "contaminated" objects.

## Guidelines for Setting Up Imaginal Exposures

Use the following strategies to create optimally effective imaginal exposures:

- **Use present tense.** Ask your client to write the imaginal exposure script using the present tense. This will have the most powerful impact when the client is reading or listening to it.

- **Include all five senses.** Have your client include as many senses as possible in the imaginal exposure script. For example, if your client has PTSD as a result of a motor vehicle accident, you should encourage him to thoroughly describe the sights (e.g., people rushing over to help, big red fire trucks in the distance), the smells (e.g., smoke, gasoline), the sensations (e.g., fear, heart racing, sweating), the sounds (e.g., hearing the ambulance sirens), and the tastes (e.g., salty blood in the mouth).

- **Include thoughts and feelings.** In addition to involving all five senses, have the client include details about the emotions, physiological sensations, and thoughts that he is experiencing. In our example of a client with PTSD from a motor vehicle accident, include physiological sensations such as pain or dizziness, emotions such as fear, and thoughts such as *I'm going to die.*

- **Include all the scary parts.** Clients may skirt around the hardest parts of the story. Ask your client up front to write down the things that would be hardest to include in a story, or the parts of the story that he would be most afraid to hear. Once the list is created, you can say, "What do you think is best for beating your fear? Should we leave all these components of the story out, or should we make sure we include them in our story?" With the psychoeducation you've already provided, your client will usually recognize and understand the importance of moving forward with the story by including the most difficult aspects.

- **Work on the story a few sentences at a time.** You can ask your client how he wants to start off the story and help him think about the general flow of it. He can write a few sentences and then read it aloud to you, giving you a chance to help edit it. Sometimes, clients will skip through the scary part, won't write it in the present tense, or won't be very descriptive, which is why we encourage you to help the client refine the story and pause after every few sentences so that you have a chance to look it over. It can be helpful to sit at a computer together and do this, which makes editing easier.

- **Don't wrap up the story on a nice note.** If a client has a fear of flying, for example, you should encourage him to end the story as the plane is going down, rather than as the plane is landing smoothly on the runway, to best target the fear.

## Exposure to Thoughts

Exposure to thoughts can be very helpful for individuals with intrusive obsessions. Just as with in vivo or imaginal exposure, in which we ask a client to face feared objects, situations, or activities, we want our clients to confront feared thoughts (as opposed to avoiding them).

### Examples of Exposure to Thoughts

Consider a client who has upsetting and repetitive thoughts such as *I have undiagnosed cancer*. The client will often try to push these thoughts out of his head or try to reassure himself that he really does not have cancer. The goal of this exposure exercise would be to repeatedly think, write, or say aloud the scariest thoughts (e.g., *I will die of cancer*) in order to confront the fear and ultimately reduce distress in the long term.

Some other examples of exposure to thoughts include:

- Deliberately thinking blasphemous, "sinful," or personally repugnant thoughts

- Deliberately thinking of "bad" words, mental images, phrases, or numbers

### Guidelines for Setting up Exposures to Thoughts

Generate a list of feared phrases or sentences that your client finds anxiety provoking. Some clients will initially be hesitant to share all of their scary thoughts with you, so ask follow-up questions, such as "Is that the scariest thought, or is there an even scarier thought than the one you just mentioned?" Once you have this list, you can ask the client to choose a feared sentence, such as "I have undetected cancer and will die," and to think about or repeat this phrase aloud. To make exposure to thoughts even more challenging later on, consider pairing these exposures with images you can find online, such as a photograph of someone who looks sick or a picture of a gravestone.

Here is an example of how to begin an exposure to feared thoughts. In this case, the client is dealing with uncomfortable thoughts related to illness anxiety disorder.

*Therapist:*    You've mentioned that you've really been struggling with some scary thoughts related to having an undiagnosed medical condition, like cancer.

*Client:*    Yes, I have been concerned that this red mark on my arm is the beginning of skin cancer. I just noticed it last week and it has been on my mind nonstop.

*Therapist:*    What do you do when these thoughts pop into your mind?

*Client:*    I try to reassure myself that I do not have skin cancer and that everything is fine. I often ask my spouse if I am okay, or I will look up what skin cancer looks like online. I sometimes do this for hours. I hate thinking these thoughts and want to stop having them.

*Therapist:*    Let's try something, just for an experiment. For a couple of minutes, I'd like you to try not to think about elephants. Okay? I'll time you. Whatever happens, don't think about elephants. (Two minutes pass.) Okay, what did you notice?

*Client:*    I tried not to think about elephants. I tried going over my grocery list instead, to keep my mind occupied. But an image of an elephant kept popping up in my mind.

*Therapist:*    I'm not surprised. It turns out that none of us is very good at that task. The reason is that the more we try to push thoughts out of our heads, the more the thoughts just pop back in. So we have to do the opposite. Instead of trying not to think these scary thoughts, we are going to face your fears by writing about, thinking about, and even saying aloud these feared thoughts. We will do this until the thoughts don't seem as scary to you anymore.

## Exposure to Bodily Sensations (Interoceptive Exposure)

Clients with various anxiety disorders, particularly (but not limited to) panic disorder and agoraphobia, often report experiencing uncomfortable physiological sensations. These sensations can include dizziness, sweating, or racing heart. Often, the client finds these sensations to be frightening. For example, instead of simply noticing that his heart is racing, the client may interpret this sensation as a catastrophic event, such as a heart attack. Just as we would ask a client to approach a feared external stimulus, we ask him to face feared *internal* stimuli, a procedure known as *interoceptive exposure*.

### Examples of Interoceptive Exposure

Interoceptive exposure can be a key component of treatment, certainly for clients with panic and agoraphobia, but also for those with other disorders, such as social anxiety disorder, OCD, or illness anxiety disorder. Some examples of interoceptive exposures include:

- Experiencing dizziness by shaking one's head repeatedly from side to side, spinning in a swivel chair, or turning in circles

- Experiencing lightheadedness or paresthesias (tingling sensations often felt in extremities or in the face) by hyperventilating

- Experiencing increased heart rate or sweating by running in place or running up a flight of stairs

- Experiencing difficulty breathing by holding one's breath, deliberately hyperventilating, or breathing through a cocktail straw

- Experiencing a stomachache by wearing a tight belt around the stomach, or by maintaining a half-sit-up until abdominal muscles fatigue

- Experiencing feelings of unreality (depersonalization or derealization) by staring at oneself in a mirror, being in a room with a strobe light, or staring at light coming through a venetian blind

- Experiencing nausea by smelling a "nausea jar" consisting of spoiled milk or meat, cigarette butts, or other foul-smelling objects

## Guidelines for Setting up Interoceptive Exposures

Designing and implementing interoceptive exposures requires careful design and implementation. First, provide information to the client about the rationale for engaging in these anxiety-provoking exercises. If you have a client who has certain medical conditions that could be exacerbated by the exercises, such as asthma, epilepsy, or heart disease, seek clearance from his medical provider prior to this intervention (refer to chapter 6 for an example of a medical clearance form).

Here is an example of how to begin interoceptive exposure with a client for the first time. In this example, the client has panic disorder and agoraphobia.

*Therapist:* Just as we have discussed ways in which we can start limiting your avoidance of feared situations, such as going into crowded stores or riding the subway, to help face your fears through exposure, we are going to begin using another type of exposure, called "interoceptive exposure." This is just a fancy way of saying that we will try to bring on those bodily sensations that you really don't like and have been trying to avoid.

*Client:* Yes, I get panicky all the time. I hate these feelings and wish they would go away. Why do we have to make them happen on purpose?

*Therapist:* Well, as you have mentioned in the past, you spend a lot of time trying to push those feelings away, either by distracting yourself or taking medication to make them go away. We want to practice bringing them on and not doing anything to make them go away. Just like other types of exposure, the more we practice, the easier it will become. I will demonstrate all of these exercises for you so that you know exactly what to do.

*Client:* What if I have a panic attack?

*Therapist:* The goal of the exposure is not to bring on a panic attack, though it is possible that one could occur. If it does, it will be a good opportunity for us to practice riding out those feelings until they settle down all on their own without engaging in any safety behaviors.

Some therapists, particularly those with a touch of exposophobia, will "water down" the interoceptive exposure intervention by taking excessively long breaks between exposures or trying to calm the client using breathing or relaxation strategies after the interoceptive exposure (Deacon, Lickel, Farrell, Kemp, & Hipol, 2013). We recommend against the use of such "calming" strategies, preferring instead to deliver the interoceptive exposure fairly intensely, which leads to superior reductions in fear (Deacon, Kemp, et al., 2013). In our practice, we do an exercise, discuss the exercise and its effects with the client for a minute or less, then start the exercise again. In order to optimize inhibitory learning (see more about this below), it's important that the client feel the sensations that he fears will lead to a heart attack, going "crazy," and so on, and recognize that these things don't happen.

We have included most of our interoceptive exposure ideas in chapter 6 of this book, as you are most likely to use interoceptive exposures with clients with panic and agoraphobia. However, these exercises can be used with any of the anxiety and related disorders in which the client is fearful of his own body sensations. Here is a typical progression of a first session of interoceptive exposure:

1.   Go through the list of interoceptive exposure ideas, which are located in chapter 6, to see which ones might be most appropriate to target your client's feared sensations. Demonstrate to the client how to do the first exercise, such as voluntary hyperventilation, and then have him do it once.

2.   Ask about the sensations that the client feels as well as the anxiety that he experienced. Then ask the client to rate the sensations and anxiety (see more on rating using SUDS below).

3.   Go to the second interoceptive exposure, show the client how to do it, and then have him do it once and rate the sensations and anxiety levels. Continue this process with the other exposures until the client has attempted each one once.

4.   Ask your client which exercise(s) he found most distressing and which ones didn't create much anxiety at all (you can let go of those).

5.   Return to an exposure that elicited moderately scary sensations as a good starting point. For example, if running in place to create a sensation of a pounding heart is where you and your client agree to start, then have the client repeat that until his fear has been reduced or he reports a sense of increased mastery over the exercise.

6.   Move on to the next item on the list.

The goal is for your client to learn that these sensations are tolerable and eventually lessen in intensity with no catastrophic consequence, thus contradicting his negative expectancies about harm (more about the principle of expectancy violation later in this chapter). Do not build in safety behaviors or give excessive reassurance to your client that he will be okay, that the anxiety will only last a few minutes, or that you are sure it is safe; these reassurances will weaken the exercises and make it less likely that the client will be able to do them on his own later without you present. Refrain, as much as possible, from stopping the exercise early due to the client's anxiety. Assign these exercises for homework so that the client can practice them without having you as a safety net. We recommend that you hold off on assigning new interoceptive exposure exercises for homework until after the client has practiced them with you in session.

## Exposures Using Virtual Reality

Virtual reality exposure therapy (VRET) is another way to help clients face and work though their fears. This approach has documented efficacy (Parsons & Rizzo, 2008). A meta-analysis of virtual reality exposure in anxiety disorders found that clients prefer VRET over some kinds of traditional in vivo exposure (Powers & Emmelkamp, 2008).

### Examples of Virtual Reality Exposures

Virtual reality exposures can be used for situations in which in vivo exposure is not possible. Some examples of VRET include:

- Simulated flights on an airplane

- Simulated speeches in front of an audience

- Simulated high places, such as walking across a bridge

- Simulated thunderstorms

- Simulated scenes from Iraq, Afghanistan, Vietnam, or 9/11

### Guidelines for Setting Up Virtual Reality Exposures

VRET does not have to be solely used for hierarchy items that cannot be recreated in session (e.g., a storm). It can also be a lower-level exposure for a client in the same way that you would use pictures of feared outcomes or online videos to help the client prior to an in vivo exposure; this is just a more realistic option. It may be very costly to have clients take repeated airplane flights to work on their fear of flying. However, through VRET, clients can take several "flights" in a row, and to make it different each time, several variables can be changed, such as the weather, time sitting on the runway, turbulence, and even whether or not they are sitting next to someone in the airplane. The graphics on many of the virtual reality devices are pretty remarkable and have come a long way since their inception.

While some good virtual reality (VR) equipment is very expensive, there are other more affordable options as well. Newer technology includes I AM Cardboard and the more advanced Google Daydream View (just one option of many), which is a headset that can be used with a variety of cell phones by downloading specific apps. Clients with a fear of spiders can see creepy, crawly spiders in front of them, and those with a fear of heights will have the opportunity to feel as though they are at the top of a skyscraper looking down below. You also have the option in many cases to purchase a controller so that the client can move around within the VR world. Some VR equipment can be purchased for under thirty dollars, giving you the opportunity to test it out and see if you want to purchase more advanced packages later on if you find yourself using it often with clients.

# CREATING AN EXPOSURE HIERARCHY

The first step in exposure therapy is to develop a list of exposure activities to be performed. We refer to this as an *exposure hierarchy*. Collaboratively with the client, we develop a list of objects, activities, situations, thoughts, or feelings that are not objectively dangerous but are nevertheless feared and avoided.

The subjective units of distress scale (SUDS; Wolpe, 1990) is a quick and easy way to obtain your client's anxiety ratings for the various exposures on his hierarchy of fears. The SUDS can be used as either a 0–100 or 0–10 scale (whichever you or your client prefer). It can be useful to give "anchors" to your clients to help them understand how to use the verbal rating scale. In other words, a "100" rating would be equal to what the client imagines is the worst anxiety he could experience, or a worst-case scenario. A "50" rating would be equal to experiencing significant levels of anxiety but being able to continue in the situation without leaving. A rating of "0" would be no anxiety at all.

For each item on the exposure hierarchy, we assign a value on the SUDS scale. We ask the client to rate, for each item, how uncomfortable he would be to confront each object, activity, situation, thought, or feeling. Here is a sample script of what the conversation might be like with your client:

*Therapist:*   What I'd like to do now is start to brainstorm a list of the things that would be frightening to you. Let's think about things that you'd rather avoid and that seem to set off your fears. What comes to mind for you?

*Client:*   Well, I'm afraid to go on an elevator. I use the stairs whenever I can. I'm really afraid the elevator's going to get stuck.

*Therapist:*   Okay, so riding an elevator would be scary to you. I'd like to get a sense of just how scary that would be. Let's use a number scale that goes from 0 to 100, where 0 is not scary at all and 100 is the scariest thing you've ever done, or could even imagine doing. Where would riding an elevator rank on this scale?

*Client:*   I think it would depend on whether there was someone else on the elevator with me. If someone else is there it's not quite as bad.

*Therapist:*      Ah, I see. That's an important distinction, so I'm glad you brought it up. So let's look at it both ways. What would your number be if you were to ride an elevator that had other people in it?

*Client:*      I think that would be about a 60.

*Therapist:*      Okay. Let's call that your fear level. So your fear level for riding an elevator with other people would be 60. What about doing the same thing, but by yourself?

*Client:*      That would be a lot scarier. Because I'd worry that I wouldn't be able to escape if it were just me.

*Therapist:*      Can you put a number to that fear, between 0 and 100?

*Client:*      That would be about a 90.

*Therapist:*      Okay, so really scary. What else can you think of?

*Client:*      I don't like wearing tight clothes, like turtlenecks, that make me feel like I can't breathe.

*Therapist:*      Okay, wearing a tight turtleneck would be scary. How scary, on that 0 to 100 scale?

*Client:*      That's about a 30, I guess.

*Therapist:*      Okay, less scary for that one. Let me run some additional scenarios by you. What would it be like for you to be in a very small space, like a small closet?

*Client:*      That would be really scary, but why would I do that? I don't need to be closed in a small closet in my daily life.

*Therapist:*      Just as an exposure exercise, to help you overcome your fear.

*Client:*      I think that would be really scary, like a 95. I don't think I can do that.

*Therapist:*      Understood. For now, we're just coming up with ideas. I suspect that if we start with things that are a bit easier, after a while you'll feel stronger and more able to tackle some of the harder things.

The therapist and client continue this discussion until they have exhausted the list of possible exposure exercises, as shown in Table 1 (you can find a blank version at the end of this chapter). As you can see in table 1, the client's fear is broken down into several concrete steps and ranked according to the SUDS level.

**TABLE 1.** Sample exposure hierarchy

| Exposure Hierarchy for My Fear: Enclosed spaces | |
|---|---|
| **Activity** | **SUDS (0–100)** |
| 1.  Flying in an airplane | 100 |
| 2.  Getting into the trunk of a car | 100 |
| 3.  Being enclosed in a small, dark closet | 95 |
| 4.  Riding an elevator by myself | 90 |
| 5.  Being rolled up in a carpet | 75 |
| 6.  Riding an elevator with others | 60 |
| 7.  Sitting in the back seat of a two-door car | 55 |
| 8.  Wearing a face mask | 50 |
| 9.  Sitting in a crowded movie theater | 45 |
| 10. Being in a hot, stuffy room | 40 |
| 11. Wearing a tight turtleneck | 30 |
| 12. Wearing a tight jacket | 25 |

Notice that the exposure hierarchy includes high-fear exposures that are not necessarily considered part of "normal" daily activity. The client noted, quite rightly, that there was no objective need to be enclosed in a small closet as part of daily living. The therapist pointed out (as discussed in chapter 1) that the aim of exposure therapy is not to mimic normal behavior, but rather to develop specific exercises that are designed to break through the fear. An important rule of the exposure hierarchy is that you should include the scariest exposures, even if the client doesn't feel able to do them right now.

# ONGOING ASSESSMENT USING SUDS

An important part of your work with your client is ongoing assessment. By assessing our clients carefully and repeatedly, we can determine whether they are getting better, getting worse, or staying the same. While there are many assessments that you may use to determine treatment progress, such as diagnosis-specific measures or more global measures of well-being, one of the simplest and most individualized ways to capture client progress is through the exposure hierarchy that the two of you have created. You can have your client rerate the exposures listed on the hierarchy at midtreatment and again at post-treatment (it may even be helpful to do this more often). Table 2 is an example of a hierarchy created with a client who has a fear of dogs. This hierarchy shows that while substantial progress has been made, there are a couple of items left to target at the top of the hierarchy.

**TABLE 2. Fear of dogs hierarchy**

| Exposure | Session 1 | Session 4 | Session 8 |
|---|---|---|---|
| Letting a large dog lick my face | 100 | 80 | 35 |
| Petting several dogs in an enclosed space (e.g., dog park) | 95 | 65 | 40 |
| Writing a story about being attacked by a big dog | 80 | 50 | 15 |
| Petting a large dog off leash | 75 | 50 | 20 |
| Visiting a dog park but not going inside the fenced-in area | 60 | 30 | 10 |
| Petting a small dog off leash | 50 | 20 | 15 |
| Petting a small dog on leash | 40 | 10 | 0 |

We do not recommend that you let your clients review or see their hierarchy ratings prior to the rerating as that could influence their ratings, so read each item aloud and ask the client for the SUDS rating and then put it into the rating sheet you have created. Clients usually enjoy seeing their progress, so you can chart their progress in a computerized document and give them a printout at posttreatment while you are reviewing their outcome in treatment. Clients are often surprised to see how high their ratings were at session 1 since so many of the exposure items are no longer problematic for them!

# HOW MUCH FEAR ARE WE AIMING FOR?

In any given exposure session, the goal is not to torture the client and make him experience sheer terror. Doing so is not only likely to be unproductive, but it also exposes the client to an unnecessary level of discomfort and increases the risk of noncompliance or dropout. On the other hand, if fear is too low during exposures, the client doesn't get a chance to benefit from the inhibitory learning (more on that in a bit) that occurs during exposure: the brain adjusting to new facts about the feared stimulus. Our preference is to have exposures be *challenging but manageable:* scary enough that new learning can take place, but not so scary that the client feels out of control. So, if the client's SUDS level is quite low, that's a sign that you have started too low on the exposure hierarchy and you should try a higher-ranked item. On the other hand, if the client's fear level is extremely high, that's a sign that you may have started too high and you need to start with something easier. In this manner, the client's fear level serves as a guide, allowing you to keep exposures in the "challenging but manageable" zone.

## HABITUATION IN EXPOSURE: IS IT NEEDED?

Aiming for habituation within a therapy session may not be as important as was once thought. Previously, it was thought that the goal of each exposure therapy session should be to promote *habituation,* or a decrease in subjective distress (see Foa & Kozak, 1986). As an example, clients would be encouraged to continue engaging in the exposure until their SUDS levels decreased by at least 50%. For instance, if a client had an initial rating of 80, then he would continue to do the exposure again and again and again until reporting a rating of 40 or less. It has been established that habituation experienced during the session, called *within-session habituation,* is not a good predictor of outcome (Craske et al., 2008)—that is, even clients whose SUDS levels don't decrease significantly during the session may still have a good response to the treatment. Of much greater importance is *between-session habituation:* the degree to which a given exposure becomes easier the next time the client tries it. Therefore, we de-emphasize within-session habituation here and talk more about watching for improvement across sessions.

## HOW LONG SHOULD EXPOSURES BE?

As noted previously, earlier versions of exposure therapy were based on the principle of within-session habituation. It was therefore believed that exposures must be prolonged, in order to allow fear to subside considerably before terminating the exposure. Indeed, early research with analogue subjects suggested that brief exposures were less effective than were longer exposures; some were also concerned that short exposures could actually make the problem worse by *sensitizing* the client to the feared stimulus (Chaplin & Levine, 1981; Stone & Borkovec, 1975). Studies with clients who have anxiety-related disorders, however, have not provided strong support for these ideas (see Craske et al., 2008). In fact, research suggests that exposure therapy might be effective even when exposures are short (e.g., Nacasch et al., 2015). In light of this research, we do not rigidly insist that all exposures be particularly long. As a rough guide, we tend to look for some evidence that inhibitory learning is taking place—a decrease in reported fear, or some degree of cognitive change (e.g., increased statements of self-efficacy)—before terminating the exposure.

# COPING DURING EXPOSURE

Recall from our discussion of exposophobia (chapter 1) that extensive coping skill training is not always necessary during exposure therapy. Though some clients (e.g., those with recurrent self-injurious behavior or other particular hazards) might benefit from emotional coping skill training prior to exposure, we find that most of our clients do not.

## Does Relaxation Help or Hurt?

It used to be thought that exposure was most effective when paired with a relaxation exercise that reduced physiological arousal. That form of exposure, called *systematic desensitization* (Wolpe, 1961), was based on the notion of "counterconditioning": whereas the feared stimulus is currently associated with a feared consequence, by associating it with relaxation, we can create a new association between the feared stimulus and a pleasant sensation. However, subsequent dismantling studies (e.g., Agras et al., 1971) demonstrated that the relaxation didn't add to the effects of exposure by itself. That is, exposure without relaxation appears to be just as effective as exposure with relaxation. In fact, in some cases (for example, clients with panic disorder), it may be that relaxation training even *detracts* from the effects of exposure: when clients were randomized to receive interoceptive and in vivo exposure, with or without a relaxing breathing training, those receiving exposure alone actually did better than did those who received exposure plus the breathing training (Schmidt et al., 2000).

How could relaxation detract from the effects of exposure, at least in the case of panic disorder? One possibility is that the relaxation exercise came to be used as a *safety behavior*. As we discussed in chapter 1, safety behaviors are those behaviors, often subtle, that make the person feel better or safer but undermine the effects of exposure by teaching a lesson of *conditional safety* (Otto et al., 2011): "I'm safe *if*...I do my relaxation exercise." We ultimately want to teach the client a lesson of *unconditional safety* in which he understands "I'm safe" without the "if."

## Do Short-Acting Medications Help or Hurt?

A parallel process may occur with the use of as-needed (or prn) short-acting benzodiazepine medications. Some evidence suggests that clients with panic disorder who take prn medications along with exposure fare less well than do clients who receive exposure alone, or who take the same medications but on a fixed dose (Westra, Stewart, & Conrad, 2002). Our theory is that the prn medication in that study taught the conditional safety message "I'm safe *if*...I take my pills," which undermined the desired unconditional safety lesson "I'm safe." In one study, clients with claustrophobia received exposure therapy along with a placebo pill. Some of the clients were told that the pill was a sedating drug that would make exposure easier; others were told either that the drug would make exposure more difficult or that it was a placebo. Although all clients did comparably well with exposure therapy in the short term, at a one-week follow-up, over a third of the group who believed they were taking a drug that would make exposure easier showed a return of their fear, compared with 0% of clients who knew they were taking a placebo (Powers, Smits, Whitley, Bystritsky, & Telch, 2008).

Conversely, exposure therapy seems to work best when there is significant *activation* of fear, rather than *deactivation* of fear. In one illustrative study of clients with PTSD who received imaginal exposure, those who exhibited more facial expression of fear benefited more from the treatment than did those who exhibited less fear (Foa, Riggs, Massie, & Yarczower, 1995). Similarly, among clients with claustrophobia, higher heart rate at the beginning of exposures predicted better outcomes of exposure therapy (Alpers & Sell, 2008). Though not all studies have replicated this result (e.g., Meuret, Seidel, Rosenfield, Hofmann, & Rosenfield, 2012; van Minnen & Hagenaars, 2002), our general sense is that clients must experience at least some degree of within-session fear activation in order for exposure therapy to be successful. In support of that notion, it has been demonstrated that when exposure therapy is combined with drugs that increase sympathetic nervous system activity (i.e., create more feelings of anxiety and tension), it produces better effects than when exposure therapy is combined with placebo or with drugs that decrease sympathetic nervous system activity (Berman & Dudai, 2001; Cain, Blouin, & Barad, 2003).

## The Art of Doing Nothing

So how do we coach our clients to cope with their distress during exposure therapy, given the fact that (for the average client) relaxing exercises and medications seem to be ineffective at best, and counterproductive at worst? We favor teaching clients *the art of doing nothing*. Individuals with anxiety disorders often overemphasize the deleterious effects of feeling fear: they worry that if they become very anxious then they will have a heart attack, go crazy, or just feel bad forever. We want to demonstrate, through experience, that this is not true. We therefore emphasize *distress tolerance* as an important skill to practice (Craske et al., 2008): in essence, coping with anxiety by not doing anything. By doing nothing in the face of anxiety, the client learns, *I can experience anxiety without it being the end of the world, and I don't necessarily have to try to make myself feel better.*

# USING THE INHIBITORY LEARNING APPROACH IN EXPOSURE WORK

In recent years, exposure therapy researchers have emphasized the principles of inhibitory learning (Craske et al., 2008; Craske, Treanor, Conway, Zbozinek, & Vervliet, 2014). In many anxiety-related disorders, fear is based on associations between a conditioned stimulus (CS) and an unconditioned stimulus (US). For example, the sight of a dog could be a CS (the stimulus the person is reacting to), and a painful bite from a dog could be a US (the consequence that the person fears will occur—whether or not it has ever actually happened to the client). Learned fear, such as that seen in anxiety-related disorders, is present when the person's reaction to the CS is similar to his reaction to the US. In this case, the person's reaction to a dog (fear) is similar to how he would react to a bite. The brain has learned to associate the CS and US, and they have come to elicit a similar response. We see this in many of our clients:

- A client with a fear of flying reacts to air travel (CS) with fear, as if it were a plane crash (US).

- A client with social phobia reacts to benign social situations (CS) with fear, as if they were humiliations (US).

- A client with OCD reacts to a public restroom (CS) with fear, as if it were covered with deadly germs (US).

So in each case, what we see is that learning has taken place: our clients have learned to respond to a relatively benign stimulus as if it were something truly dangerous or threatening. During the course of exposure therapy, the CS is presented repeatedly without the US (we call this a *CS-noUS pairing*). In the case of a dog fear, as just one example, we present the dog without the bite. Over the course of exposure, the fear response is *extinguished:* The person no longer "confuses" dogs with bites and can respond to a friendly dog without feelings of fear.

What's happening during this process, at a neurobiological level, is that the prefrontal cortical (PFC) regions of the brain start to inhibit regions of the limbic system such as the amygdala (Delgado, Nearing, Ledoux, & Phelps, 2008). Though the initial CS-US pairing isn't necessarily eliminated from long-term memory, these new CS-noUS associations become the dominant response—a process known as *inhibitory learning.* It's called "inhibitory" because one process in the brain is inhibiting another. Our job as therapists is to get the PFC regions to be as active as possible, so that we maximize CS-noUS learning. Below, we will discuss several of these strategies that may help clients develop and retrieve nonthreat associations.

## Maximizing Expectancy Violation

Rescorla and Wagner's (1972) learning theory suggests that the success of extinction is the result of a *mismatch* between clients' expectations about what they believe will happen and what they actually experience. Our job as therapists is to maximize the client's experience of "surprise" during an exposure. We can do this by ensuring that exposures are long enough to violate the expectancy. Earlier theorists (e.g., Foa & Kozak, 1986) recommended long exposures to allow sufficient time for within-session habituation—that is, long enough for the client's anxiety to diminish significantly during the exposure. However, as noted by Craske et al. (2008), clinical research raises questions about the necessity of long exposures and within-session habituation for fear reduction. In one study, the length of exposure did not seem to matter, as long as there was sufficient time for *expectancy violation*—that is, as long as the exposure was long enough for the client to be surprised (Baker et al., 2010).

In the following example, the therapist seeks to maximize expectancy violation by focusing on surprises and cognitive change. The therapist and client (who has panic disorder) have just completed an interoceptive exposure exercise involving running in place.

*Therapist:*   Okay, we've been running for one minute. Let's pause now. What physical sensations are you noticing?

*Client:*   Well, I definitely notice that my heart is racing, and I feel shortness of breath. And I feel a little sweaty.

*Therapist:*   And how similar are these feelings to what you experience when you're panicky? Let's use a scale from 0 to 10, where 0 is not at all like what you experience, and 10 is exactly what you experience.

*Client:*   It's definitely similar; I'd say an 8.

*Therapist:*   Okay. And what's your SUDS level? That's our 0 to 100 scale of how scary it is.

*Client:*   I'd say about a 70.

*Therapist:*   Okay, so pretty scary. Did your brain tell you something scary about this exercise? Like that something bad was going to happen?

*Client:*   Yeah, it told me I was going to have a panic attack and freak out.

*Therapist:*   It does that a lot, doesn't it? Let's just experience these sensations for a moment and pay attention to what happens. What, if anything, surprised you about this exercise?

*Client:*   I guess I was mostly surprised by the fact that I didn't panic.

*Therapist:*   So what's the lesson learned here? What information do you want your brain to absorb?

*Client:*   That just because my heart's racing, that doesn't mean I'm going to panic.

*Therapist:*   Exactly. You're teaching your brain that your heart can race, and that doesn't have to be a big deal. You did a really nice job with that exercise. Let's keep it up!

## Limiting Distraction

It is important for the client to limit the use of distraction during exposure therapy. Research generally suggests that it is more beneficial to be focused on the exercise or exposure, including paying attention to the feared situation and the feeling of fear in the body, as opposed to trying to distract from it (Grayson, Foa, & Steketee, 1982; Kamphuis & Telch, 2000; Telch et al., 2004). Distraction can have several negative effects on exposure. First, it breaks up the exposure, so that instead of one long exposure session, the client is actually experiencing several briefer exposure sessions (which are potentially not long enough to violate expectancies, as discussed above), punctuated by periods of distracted attention. Second, distraction impairs the client's ability to recognize that the disaster is not occurring in the presence of the feared situation or stimulus. You need to be on the lookout for distraction in your clients and need to help bring them back to the exposure if they start to go off course. In this example, the therapist is working with a client who has a fear of elevators.

*Therapist:*  Okay, we are on the elevator and are going to continue to ride it up and down the ten floors like we previously agreed, to target your fear of getting stuck. I want you to focus on what you see in the elevator and how you feel without engaging in any distractions.

*Client:*  Okay. (A few moments go by.) I forgot to tell you earlier that I had difficulty with some of the therapy homework you gave me last week and I have some questions about it.

*Therapist:*  We can definitely address this following the exposure. Right now, I would like you to try to stick with this exposure without thinking about other things since it is considered distraction. To come back into the exposure, think about the way the elevator feels moving up and down, what the buttons look like, how your heart is racing, and so on. Let's stand quietly for the rest of the ride.

## Fear-Antagonistic Actions

It can be useful to encourage the client to engage in *fear-antagonistic actions*—that is, behaving as if he is unafraid (Weisman & Rodebaugh, 2018). Research demonstrates that exposure therapy is more effective when clients are instructed to engage in "brave" behaviors, such as running toward the balcony for those with fear of heights (Wolitzky & Telch, 2009) or deliberately stuttering during a speech for those with public speaking fears (Nelson, Deacon, Lickel, & Sy, 2010). These actions serve to maximize the mismatch between expectancies (for example, stuttering during a speech and everyone laughing and pointing at him) and outcomes (stuttering on purpose during a speech and the audience not reacting poorly). In this example, the therapist is working with a client who has a fear of heights, and they are standing on a high balcony together.

*Therapist:*  You're doing a great job with this exposure. I'm really impressed that you got up here.

*Client:*  Yeah, I feel like it's getting easier the more time we spend up here.

*Therapist:*   I wonder whether we could up the ante a little bit. Right now I notice that you're backed away from the railing and are being very still.

*Client:*      That's true; I am. I guess I'm still feeling kind of nervous.

*Therapist:*   That's completely understandable. But what I'd like to have you do is act as if you were completely unafraid. Let's think about that for a moment. If you were completely unafraid, what would you be doing up here?

*Client:*      Um, I guess I'd be closer to the railing?

*Therapist:*   Yes, probably. How would you get to the railing, if you were completely unafraid? Would you tiptoe toward it?

*Client:*      No, I guess I would just walk up to it.

*Therapist:*   I wonder whether we could even take that a little further and have you walk very quickly toward the railing?

*Client:*      That would be really scary. I'd worry that I would fall over.

*Therapist:*   Yes, I could imagine that's what your brain would be telling you. But perhaps we don't need to listen to that part of your brain right now. Perhaps we could just act completely unafraid and walk really briskly over to the railing, like this (demonstrates). Now can you try that?

*Client:*      I guess I can try. (Client walks briskly to the railing.)

*Therapist:*   Great job. Now let's really act unafraid. Can we run over toward the railing, like this (demonstrates)?

*Client:*      Wow, that just seems really scary. I think if I did that, I would fall right over.

*Therapist:*   You think you wouldn't be able to stop. But is that really true? Has anything like that ever actually happened to you?

*Client:*      No, I guess not.

*Therapist:*   No. That's just your brain trying to talk you out of this. But let's show your fear who's boss by running right up to the railing.

*Client:*      Okay, I can try it.

## Deepened Extinction

The concept of "deepened extinction" (Rescorla, 2006) refers to the simultaneous presentation of multiple CSs, which have previously been extinguished in isolation or though one part of the hierarchy at a time. When multiple feared stimuli are presented at the same time ("piled on"), we maximize the client's ability to be surprised by the outcome. For example, if a client has PTSD from being mugged in an alleyway, you may have helped him do various exposures to target this fear, such as reading stories of others who were mugged, going to new alleyways, and eventually going back to the scene of the incident. When you are piling on stimuli at the same time (usually in later therapy sessions), you may ask the client to visit the alleyway while also reading aloud a story about being mugged.

Here, the therapist is working with a client who has panic disorder and agoraphobia. In previous sessions, they have conducted interoceptive exposures, including hyperventilating and spinning. Today, the therapist and client are meeting in a crowded shopping mall and have spent some time walking through the crowd.

*Therapist:* You've done a nice job tolerating the distress of being here in the mall. I can see that you feel a little more comfortable with it.

*Client:* Yeah, I feel okay. It's still kind of scary, but I'm handling it a bit.

*Therapist:* What I'd like to do now is combine this exposure—walking through the mall—with an exposure that we've already done. Do you remember a couple of weeks ago when we practiced hyperventilating in my office?

*Client:* Yeah, I got really lightheaded and nauseated.

*Therapist:* Yes, and then you started to feel less fearful, right?

*Client:* Yes, I did.

*Therapist:* So what I'd like to do now is have you hyperventilate here in the mall. Here's my thinking behind that: Right now, you're doing a great job tolerating the distress of being in the mall, and you feel okay physically. What we need to do next is have you practice tolerating the discomfort of being in the mall even when you don't feel okay physically. So I want us to practice feeling bad in the mall so that your brain starts to learn that's not a threat either. Does that make sense?

*Client:* Yes, I guess so. It's a scary idea, though.

*Therapist:* Yes, and that's all the more reason why we should tackle this fear and make sure that the mall can't scare you, even when you don't feel okay. So can we do some hyperventilating right here, together?

*Client:* Okay. (They hyperventilate.)

*Therapist:* Perfect. What's your fear level right now?

*Client:* About an 80. It's scary.

*Therapist:* Okay, so let's just walk around now and see how this feels.

## Eliminating Safety Behaviors

Safety behaviors are subtle (and sometimes not so subtle) things that the client does to feel safer. The most obvious example of safety behaviors are compulsions (e.g., hand washing, ordering, checking) exhibited by clients with OCD, though safety behaviors can be seen in any of the anxiety and related disorders. When safety behaviors are used during an exposure (for example, a client with OCD washing his hands, a client with panic disorder carrying an anxiolytic medication, or a client with social anxiety standing in an empty corner at a party), the nonoccurrence of the US is attributed not to the *unconditional safety* of the situation, but to the *conditional safety* of the behavior. In other words, safety behaviors contribute to learning things like "I'm safe *if*…I wash my hands when they appear dirty."

Several studies show that exposure efficacy is improved when anxious clients are discouraged from engaging in safety behaviors (Hedtke, Kendall, & Tiwari, 2009; Kim, 2005; Powers, Smits, & Telch, 2004; Sloan & Telch, 2002). Conversely, some analogue (student) samples have failed to replicate this finding (Deacon, Sy, Lickel, & Nelson, 2010; Levy & Radomsky, 2014; Rachman, Shafran, Radomsky, & Zysk, 2011). Our opinion, based on all of the available data, is that safety behaviors are often (though not always) detrimental to the process of exposure therapy, and there is little evidence to suggest that they are helpful (at least in clients with anxiety disorders).

In this example, the therapist is coaching a client with panic disorder on a homework assignment to ride a city bus.

*Therapist:* One thing that's really important is to get rid of all of those things, big or little, that you do to try to feel better, or that you think might be keeping you safe. What kinds of things can you envision having with you on the bus that would fit that description?

*Client:* Definitely my bottle of pills. I don't even take them that much, but just having the bottle makes me feel a lot better.

*Therapist:* Understood. The problem we run into is that anxiety is really good at saying "I'm safe if…" and then putting all of these rules around what's safe and what's not safe. And of course, the problem is that one of these days you're going to find yourself in a tight situation without your pills, and your brain won't have learned that that situation is safe, too. Does that make sense?

*Client:* Yes, I understand that, but it's a lot scarier to ride the bus if I don't have my pills with me.

*Therapist:* It makes sense that that would be scarier for you. You've relied on these pills for a long time, like a crutch. But we know that exposure therapy is going to work a lot better for you if you don't bring your crutch with you.

*Client:* So I should leave my pills at home when I ride the bus.

*Therapist:* Exactly.

# Occasional Reinforced Extinction

Occasional reinforced extinction refers to occasionally allowing the CS and US to be paired during exposure (Woods & Bouton, 2007). This may seem clinically counterintuitive, as we generally think that exposure works when the CS is presented repeatedly in the *absence* of the US. However, it can sometimes be helpful to arrange for the "disaster" to occur during exposure. Our experience has been that exposure to certain "disasters," when handled carefully, can serve to diminish the threat value of the US, which can teach the client that even if the "disaster" occurs, the results are not necessarily catastrophic. For example, for the client with social anxiety disorder who fears making audience members bored during a presentation, you may set up an audience of confederates (e.g., trainees or colleagues) and ask some of them to scroll through their phones, yawn, or even leave the presentation early. This will set up the "disaster" for the client in order to help him get through the worst-case scenario and live through it. Here, the therapist is working with a client with OCD who has a fear that she will harm others by having bad thoughts about them.

*Therapist:*  For our next exposure, I wonder whether you could wish for me to develop a brain tumor.

*Client:*  That's scary, but I can try.

*Therapist:*  Okay, so wish for that out loud: "I wish for you to get a brain tumor."

*Client:*  I wish for you to get a brain tumor.

*Therapist:*  What's your level now?

*Client:*  About a 60.

*Therapist:*  Okay, so that's not so bad. The next thing I'd like to try is that you wish for me to get a brain tumor, but this time I'm going to tell you whether I feel anything.

*Client:*  Okay. I wish for you to get a brain tumor.

*Therapist:*  I'm feeling a slight headache at the moment.

*Client:*  Yeah, that's scary.

*Therapist:*  What's your fear level?

*Client:*  That's an 80.

*Therapist:*  Okay, let's stay with this exposure for a bit. You keep wishing for me to get a brain tumor, and I'll keep describing my headache to you.

## Changing the Context

Fear can be reinstated after extinction if the context in which the individual encounters the feared stimulus changes (Mineka, Mystkowski, Hladek, & Rodriguez, 1999); this phenomenon can be lessened by conducting exposure in multiple contexts (Bouton, 1993). Varying the kind of exposures conducted—for example, exposure to several different kinds of dogs, rather than one kind—is one straightforward way of increasing variability, thereby reducing the likelihood that fear will return. Another is to change the conditions under which the client encounters the stimulus. For example, we could vary the *external* contexts by conducting exposures in the therapist's office, outside, and in the patient's home or other location, during the day and at night. We could also vary the *internal* context by having the patient engage in exposures both when relatively calm and after fear has been aroused.

In this example, the therapist is working with a client who has panic disorder and agoraphobia. Having completed a session of interoceptive exposure in the session, the therapist now assigns in vivo exposure homework.

*Therapist:*   Last week, you went to the mall and walked through the crowds, and you did a really great job with it. I'm interested in having you do something similar, but changing the context a bit. Are there some other really crowded places you could go to besides the mall?

*Client:*   Hmm. I guess maybe a sporting event of some kind? I used to like to go to ball games, but I stopped going because of the crowds.

*Therapist:*   That's a really good idea. What would you think of trying to get to a ball game this week?

## CONCLUSIONS

In this chapter, we have reviewed the various types of exposures that can be useful in helping your clients face their fears: in vivo exposure, imaginal exposure, exposure to thoughts, interoceptive exposure, and using virtual reality in exposure. Exposure therapy is partly about what we ask the client to *do,* but it is also partly about what we ask the client *not* to do. We discussed some inhibitory learning principles as well as strategies to help clients to extinguish the association between a feared object, thought, situation, or sensation and the feared consequence.

In the next chapter, we'll talk about doing exposure with children and adolescents. We will teach you how to best work with the parents of your client as your co-therapists. In addition, we will give you advice on how to make the therapy experience easier to understand and even more engaging for your younger clients.

# CHAPTER RESOURCES

**Reminder:** These resources are also available to download and print from http://www.newharbinger.com/43737.

| Exposure Hierarchy for My Fear: | |
|---|---|
| **Activity** | **SUDS (0–100)** |
| 1. | |
| 2. | |
| 3. | |
| 4. | |
| 5. | |
| 6. | |
| 7. | |
| 8. | |
| 9. | |
| 10. | |
| 11. | |
| 12. | |
| 13. | |
| 14. | |
| 15. | |

## Interoceptive Exposure: Anxiety Tracking Using Suds

| Activity | Time 1 SUDS (0–100) | Time 2 SUDS (0–100) | Time 3 SUDS (0–100) |
|---|---|---|---|
| **Example:** Hyperventilating for 60 seconds | 70 | 55 | 35 |
| | | | |
| | | | |
| | | | |
| | | | |
| | | | |
| | | | |
| | | | |
| | | | |
| | | | |
| | | | |

# CHAPTER 4

# Helping Kids Climb the Exposure Ladder

Now that we have reviewed the rationale for exposure therapy as well as how to effectively design and implement various types of exposures (e.g., in vivo, imaginal, and interoceptive), this chapter will focus on how to work creatively and effectively with your younger clients and their parents. As mentioned in chapter 1, clinicians with exposophobia may have a misconception that children won't do well with exposure therapy. However, children can do very well with it and can often understand quite quickly why we are using it—sometimes even better than our adult clients! Many of the same principles still apply when conducting exposure with a younger population. That being said, there are some important tweaks that you can make to the treatment to help better engage the client: adapting the psychoeducation component; including the parent(s) in session; using child-friendly strategies such as naming the anxiety, drawing the anxiety "creature," playing games, and getting out of the office; and rewarding the behaviors you would like to see the child continue to do.

## PSYCHOEDUCATION WITH CHILDREN AND ADOLESCENTS

Just as with your adult clients, you want your younger clients to know what to expect in treatment and to have the opportunity to ask any questions they may have about your work with them. You are asking your clients to do the very thing they fear. This can sound scary to your younger clients (just as it can to your adult clients), but it's all in the delivery of how you explain exposure therapy to them. Here's an example of a conversation you could have with a younger client about what to expect during exposure therapy:

*Therapist:*   I'm so glad that you are going to start doing exposure therapy. We're going to work together as teammates during this time to help you feel better and get your anxiety to stop bossing you around. Does that sound okay to you?

*Client:*   Yes, but what is exposure therapy?

*Therapist:*   Let me give you an example of what therapy will look like. Do you like dogs?

*Client:*   Yes! I love dogs and even have one.

*Therapist:*    That's great! I really like dogs too. What you would do to help a friend who maybe wanted to come over to your house to play but was really scared of dogs?

*Client:*       I could put the dog in my basement so she wouldn't be afraid.

*Therapist:*    Do you think that will help your friend learn to like dogs and no longer be afraid?

*Client:*       Well, no, because she wouldn't ever see my dog so she wouldn't get to see how friendly she is.

*Therapist:*    Exactly. Hiding away or avoiding something scary doesn't help you get over your fear. So, let's think of some other things we could do to help your friend.

*Client:*       We could show her my neighbors' dog who is really small and lies around a lot so there isn't much to be scared of.

*Therapist:*    Wonderful idea. Then once your friend starts finding it easy to be around your neighbors' small dog, you could let your friend meet an even bigger dog. We might even want to think about things such as starting easy with a dog on a leash and then later having the dog be off the leash.

*Client:*       Oh, I get it. Yeah, we could even ask my friend to stand far away from the dog and then get closer to it.

*Therapist:*    Maybe as one of the very last exposures you could have your friend go with you to a dog park where there are lots of jumpy dogs.

*Client:*       That would be so scary to my friend right now.

*Therapist:*    I bet. So that's why we start off with the smaller cute puppy and work our way up the exposure ladder to more challenging exposures. This is what we are going to do every time you come to my office. I want you to help me come up with a list of things we can do together to gradually help you with your anxiety. Think you are up for the challenge?

# PARENT-BASED INTERVENTIONS

When doing exposure therapy with children, we often modify treatment to include the parents as "co-therapists" (Piacentini et al., 2011). Two particularly helpful interventions are (a) including parents in exposure therapy and (b) helping parents to reduce their reassurance-giving and other accommodations to their child's anxiety.

## Including Parents in Exposure

It can be beneficial to have the parents see what you are doing with the younger client so that they can help their child at home and act as effective co-therapists. After you have provided the parents with psychoeducation about exposure therapy and how it will be used to treat their child's anxiety, invite the parents into the room to watch an exposure session. There are several things you should go over with the parents in session so that they can continue to help their child at home. These include prompting the child to do exposure homework, coaching her through the exposure, and praising the child's hard work.

### Prompting

Younger clients may not remember to work on the problem on their own, or they may be less intrinsically motivated to change maladaptive behaviors and to face feared situations than are some adult clients. Therefore, we encourage parents to prompt the child to do her exposure homework between sessions. It can be helpful for parents to talk with their child ahead of time (or better yet, in session) to decide what time of day the child is going to work on exposure. Once a time is set up, the parents should gently remind the child that it is time to begin homework. If a predetermined time is not scheduled, the child and parents may be more likely to battle each other over homework. We suggest having the parents and/or the child set alarms on their smartphones or other devices so that they are prompted to do the exposure homework. You can ask the family to set their phone alarms when you are assigning homework for the week.

### Coaching

In addition to reminding the child to do the exposure homework, the parents can coach the child through the exposure homework assignment. Especially earlier in treatment, the parents might have a better handle on exposure, and how to implement it, than does the child. The parents can remind the child about how to start the exposure, what safety behaviors to be on the lookout for (and how to eliminate them), and when to stop the exposure.

### Praising

Encourage parents to praise their child for attempting and completing exposure exercises. The child does not always need to have a reward or treat but can benefit from the parents' verbal praise. The parents can say, "Nice work; you really fought hard to do the opposite of what your anxiety was telling you to do," "You were so brave," "That was really impressive," and "Keep up the amazing work—I know how hard this is." As a clinician it can be helpful to watch how the parents praise (or don't praise) the child in session. Model for the parent how you praise the child during or following the exposure. Don't forget to praise the parents for all of their hard work too!

## Reducing Reassurance-Giving and Other Family Accommodations

Reducing reassurance and other accommodations is an essential part of CBT for children and adolescents with anxiety and related disorders. In fact, even if the younger client refuses treatment and does not set foot into your office, this is a topic that you can address with the parents, which can trickle down to helping the child in the long run.

One of your first jobs as a therapist tackling an anxiety-related disorder in a younger client is to determine the degree of *family accommodation*: the extent to which parents or other family members have altered their own behavior to adjust for the child's fear. Explain to the family that accommodations are things that they do or say to cater to the child's fear in an attempt to make the child more comfortable. These accommodations tend to grow and get out of control over time. For example, the child with OCD may ask her parents to wash their hands before touching the family computer. The parents may initially agree to do so, so that the child can continue to use the computer and feel comfortable. However, over time the parents may start washing themselves repeatedly before touching any item in the house in the presence of the child, or even disinfecting objects within the home.

Accommodations can take many forms. Examples of commonly seen family accommodations to the child's anxiety include the following:

- Parents provide excessive reassurance to the child that things are okay or that the child will not get hurt, anxious, dirty, or kidnapped.

- Parents refrain from sending the child to needed after-school care while they are at work, or leave work early due to the child's separation fears.

- Parents buy extra soap, hand sanitizer, or other household cleaners due to the child's concern about contamination.

- Parents change clothes when entering the home to be "clean" and may even have siblings do the same.

- Parents refrain from using certain words, phrases, or sentences that elicit the child's anxiety.

Over time, parents can easily get swept up in giving reassurance and providing accommodations to their child even when the child isn't asking for it. For example, if a child with OCD is practicing touching dirty items in the therapy office, one of the parents might say, "Don't worry; that is probably not very dirty and won't hurt you," or "You can shower when you go home tonight." This is a wonderful opportunity to gently remind the parents about why such statements, though intended to be caring and helpful, are contraindicated in treatment. Let them know you don't expect all of this to change overnight and that you will work with them to remind them to make fewer reassurance statements, and give them their own homework to practice during the week as well.

Remember, there is no one to blame here. At the end of the day, the parents are just trying to make their kids feel better and to have less anxiety. The problem is that the reassurance-giving and other accommodations, such as those described above, may work as a short-term fix for the child's anxiety, but the problem doesn't get any better in the long run. Ultimately, the reassurance-giving and excessive accommodations prolong the child's anxiety. It is critical to help the parents understand the long-term consequences of these behaviors and help them learn healthier strategies. Here's an example of how to have this conversation with the parents of a child with contamination-based OCD:

*Therapist:* Now that we've talked more in depth about exposure therapy, I wanted to have a conversation with you about things we can change in order to help your daughter make the most progress she can in therapy.

*Parent:* Sure, that sounds great.

*Therapist:* You've mentioned that your daughter asks you questions over and over again even when you have already answered them; is that right?

*Parent:* Yes, she repeatedly asks all sorts of questions, such as, "Will I get sick from using my friend's pencil at school today?" and the other one we hear all the time is "Am I going to be okay?"

*Therapist:* How do you typically handle those questions?

*Parent:* First, we usually say, "You're fine; don't worry about it."

*Therapist:* Does that satisfy her and her anxiety?

*Parent:* Hardly ever anymore. Usually, she doesn't like the answer and tries to get us to say something very specific, such as "I promise that you will not get sick."

*Therapist:* Are there other accommodations you make to your child's anxiety?

*Parents:* Yes. It's become quite extensive. We feel as though we are constantly catering to her anxiety. She asks us to remove our work clothes before entering the house and will never let us enter her room or sit on her bed unless she is reassured that we are clean. We do more laundry than ever before, because she goes through so many of her clothes during the week due to her need to be clean.

*Therapist:* I see. Have you ever tried cutting back on these accommodations in the past?

*Parent:* Yes, and it went horribly. She cried, and begged, and told us we were awful parents. It was really hard to see and hear.

*Therapist:* That must have been really hard. What ended up happening after she pleaded with you?

*Parent:* Eventually we promised she wouldn't get sick or be contaminated. We did everything we could to make her feel better, even though it has been hard on us time-wise and financially.

| | |
|---|---|
| *Therapist:* | Got it. What you did is very understandable. As parents, you want to protect your child and take away negative feelings. That's really normal. But, has it helped your daughter get over her fears of touching dirty things, or alleviated her worries about getting sick? |
| *Parent:* | No, it's worse than it's ever been. |
| *Therapist:* | Okay, so it sounds like you gave it a good shot to try to eliminate her anxiety by reassuring her and accommodating the anxiety, but as you say, it hasn't helped. In this treatment, we are going to try something different. We are going to limit and eventually eliminate altogether the reassurance and other accommodations you are giving your daughter when it comes to her OCD-related fears. |
| *Parent:* | That sounds hard. |
| *Therapist:* | It is hard at first, but like anything else, it gets easier. Your child will also be prepared that this is coming, and will know why you are being asked to do this. Since the level of reassurance-seeking is pretty high right now, let's start with you being able to answer the question your daughter asks you only once, and if she asks it again you can say, "I already answered that; remember what I said before." Then don't say anything else. |
| *Parent:* | Okay, I think we can do that. |
| *Therapist:* | We will make this increasingly more challenging over time by giving no reassurance at all and then maybe even giving the opposite of the kind of reassurance your daughter is seeking. For example, your child may ask, "Will I get sick?" and I'd encourage you to answer with, "Yes, you're going to get sick." We'll make sure to give your daughter advance notice that you'll be answering questions in this way. |
| *Parent:* | That sounds so hard! |
| *Therapist:* | That will come later on in therapy, but I wanted to give you an idea of where we will be heading. By the time you are asked to do that, it likely will not be as challenging for you or your daughter as it sounds today, because you will have already done so many other things. Other examples of assignments I give you might include only doing one load of laundry per week, or limiting the soap in the house, or even eliminating it all together for a period of time. |
| *Parent:* | Okay, we can give it a try. |
| *Therapist:* | I do want you to keep in mind that the key to this working is being consistent with the assignments I give you related to cutting back on all of the accommodations related to her OCD. It won't work as well if you give reassurance sometimes, or if you give in when she begs and pleads. Are you up for committing to doing this consistently to help your daughter? |

## When Children Refuse Treatment

If you work with children or adolescents, you know that sometimes they refuse treatment even when they are struggling tremendously. This can be challenging for a family and can leave them confused about the next steps. Fortunately, you can work directly with the parents to help modify their behaviors, which will ultimately benefit the child. Parent work alone has been shown to improve outcomes, even when the child is reluctant to engage in treatment. As one example, the SPACE Program (which stands for Supportive Parenting for Anxious Childhood Emotions) is a treatment protocol designed for parents to learn new strategies and help treat child and adolescent anxiety, without the child's direct participation with the therapist (Lebowitz, 2013; Lebowitz, Omer, Hermes, & Scahill, 2014).

The younger client may be upset that you and the parents are continuing in treatment even though she has refused. Have the parents periodically invite their child to join the therapy and to add her input at any time. It is important that parents keep their child informed about treatment and what to expect, rather than changing everything up and withdrawing accommodations without giving any notice to the child.

We have included a worksheet at the end of this chapter for you to keep track of the family accommodations that are being made for the child's anxiety. You can share this worksheet with the parents, and they can add accommodations that need to be eliminated to the worksheet as well. Make sure to assign homework for the parents that includes reducing these behaviors.

# CHILD-FRIENDLY STRATEGIES

When working with children and adolescents with anxiety disorders, it's important to incorporate fun ways to engage them in the sessions. This can include playing games, drawing the anxiety monster, and getting out of the office. We'll describe child-friend approaches in greater detail below.

## Using Games to Help Kids Learn

Following psychoeducation with the parent(s) and child or adolescent, you can explore how much your young client has learned about exposure by turning it into a game. We often ask our adult clients to summarize the treatment back to us, so that we can gauge their level of understanding and correct any misconceptions. For some of our younger clients, instead of a back and forth conversation, we'll play "host" of a "game show" in which we quiz the child on some of the key psychoeducational points. Invite the parents to play the game too, to see who can buzz in the fastest and win the most points. Even if the child is getting some of the answers wrong, she is still learning. The sample Psychoeducation Game Show Questions and Answers list at the end of the chapter consists of generic questions related to CBT and exposure, but we encourage you to add more specific questions related to that child or adolescent's diagnosis. For example, if the child has panic disorder, you may want to add questions such as "True or false: Panic attacks are uncomfortable but harmless." (True).

## Naming the Anxiety

A good way to help your younger client learn to separate herself from the anxiety and to externalize it is to name it. For example, a client with OCD who lines everything up perfectly and in order might decide to name the OCD "Mr. Perfect." Then you (and the parents) can say to the child, "Is it really true that you want to spend twenty minutes lining things up just so before going out to the movies, or is that something Mr. Perfect is telling you to do?" Over time the child will learn that it is the anxiety, Mr. Perfect, who is bossing her around, telling her what she can and cannot do. This is a nice way to help the child see that she needs to "boss back" the anxiety (e.g., March & Mulle, 1998) and to do what she wants to do (e.g., go to the movies on time) without listening to Mr. Perfect's instructions.

Sometimes clients will have difficulty coming up with a name on the spot, so give them some examples of various names and assign naming the anxiety for homework. Ask your client to think about various characters from books, television shows, or movies to come up with a name for the anxiety.

Here are some examples of names that might suit your client's anxiety:

- Mr. Perfect—This is a good example of a name to describe the anxiety of someone who is very perfectionistic, hates making mistakes and avoids them at all costs, and tries to do things in exactly the "right way."

- Mr. Clean—This is a good name for a client whose OCD involves contamination fears, and who engages in cleaning rituals or tries to avoid coming into contact with objects, places, or people who are perceived to be dirty.

- Regina George—A character from the movie *Mean Girls,* Regina George is the epitome of a high school bully. She is bossy to others, manipulates them, and acts as though she is superior to those around her.

- Miss Worrywart—This is an example of a name to describe the anxiety of clients who may be engaged in excessive ruminating, obsessing, or worrying.

Let the younger client explain to her parents why she is naming the anxiety and why she chose that particular name. Encourage the parents to use the anxiety's name as well at home, and give the parents examples of how to use it. For example, if your younger client has contamination-related OCD and has been having a hard time getting out of the bathroom in the morning because she is caught up in compulsions, the parents can say, "Wow, looks like Mr. Clean (or whatever name the child has chosen) has been really bossy to you and is telling you that you can't come down for breakfast unless you wash your hands again. Do you want to let Mr. Clean keep bossing your around, or should we boss him back?"

## Drawing the Anxiety Creature

It can be helpful to encourage the child to draw a picture of the anxiety creature, so that she can hold the image in her mind of whom exactly she is fighting. This can be a good homework assignment or something that you do with your younger client in session, especially if she has been slow to warm up. If a younger child is shy about it at first, you can give her examples of characteristics to give her anxiety creature, such as a unibrow, a head of spiky hair, or green teeth. In the final session of therapy, you can make a photocopy of the child's anxiety creature and allow the child to rip it up and throw it away, signifying that she beat the anxiety creature.

## Getting Out of the Office

Exposure often involves doing work outside of the confines of the office. Ask the younger client's parent(s) to join you in leaving the office space or get permission to do so one on one with your client, such as going outside or to another floor of the building to do an exposure. We don't recommend driving with clients in your car, so when you are planning an exposure at a separate location (e.g., grocery store, mall), we suggest you meet the child and parents at the site.

# USING REWARDS

It is not always essential to use a reward system during exposure therapy with a child. Some children will be very motivated to work on the anxiety or other difficulty without needing any incentives other than verbal praise. However, you may find yourself working with a younger child who may not fully understand the rationale for exposure and therefore is more reluctant. In such cases, consider using a reward chart.

If you decide to use a reward system with your younger client, there are some guidelines we suggest you keep in mind.

## Refrain from Using Rewards as Bribes

Reward charts should be individualized to the client so that she can be working toward earning fun activities or things. Rewards need not (and should not) be expensive. They can include earning extra time on the computer or video game console or getting to choose where the family is ordering take-out food from that night. You (and the parents) are not using the reward system as a bribe to get the child to do the exposure, but rather are rewarding the child's hard work in fighting back against anxiety and taking better control of her life. Rewards should be planned ahead of time so that the child or adolescent knows exactly what she is working toward earning. Bribes, as opposed to rewards, tend to be more spontaneous in nature. Have this conversation with the parent(s) about the reward system so that they know how to best implement it at home.

## Create a Rewards Menu

When creating the reward chart, include both short-term rewards that the child could earn daily and longer-term rewards. For the latter, the child can choose to save up points and cash them in for a bigger activity or special occasion later on. We have included a list of ideas for you to consider with both the child and parent(s) when creating your chart. Brainstorm other ideas in session with both the younger client and parent(s).

### Quick-to-earn prizes

- **Skip a chore.** Choose a typical chore done at home to skip for the evening (e.g., dishes, picking up room).

- **Bonus time added to bedtime.** Go to bed fifteen (or other predetermined number) minutes later.

- **Extra screen time.** Get fifteen (or other predetermined number) extra minutes of TV time or videogame time.

- **Go outside.** Go to a nearby park or play a game outside in the yard.

### Harder-to-earn prizes

- **Sleepover.** Have a sleepover with a friend or at a family member's house.

- **Spend the day with a friend.** Have a friend over or go to a friend's house for the day.

- **Get pampered.** Get a manicure or pedicure.

- **Get a treat.** Go out for ice cream or another treat.

- **Get a new toy.** Pick out a toy or game under $20.

- **Get to choose dinner.** Choose a dinner restaurant or take-out option for the family for the night.

- **Movie date.** Go to a movie theater and choose the movie.

- **Do an activity.** Go mini-golfing or bowling.

## CONCLUSIONS

Exposure treatment for many of the anxiety-related disorders is quite effective with child and adolescent clients. As we have discussed, there are some nuances of doing successful exposure work with children and adolescents, including the importance of working with parents. Having the parents reduce their accommodations to their child's fear during exposure work, as well as having them refrain from providing their child with excessive reassurance, is critical. And by incorporating strategies such as playing games, naming the anxiety, and setting up rewards (not bribes), you can increase the likelihood that your younger clients will be motivated to engage in exposures.

Now that you are equipped with how to best design and implement exposures, with both adults and younger clients, we will start our venture into part 2 of the book, which dives deep into creative and effective exposure ideas. The chapters in part 2 are dedicated to each of the anxiety and related disorders for which you are most likely to use exposure as *the* treatment or as a major component of the treatment.

## CHAPTER RESOURCES

**Reminder:** These resources are also available to download and print from http://www. newharbinger.com/43737.

## List of Accommodations to Be Eliminated

| Accommodation | Difficulty level (1–100) |
|---|---|
| **Example:** Giving reassurance that everything will be okay | 85 |
| | |
| | |
| | |
| | |
| | |
| | |
| | |
| | |
| | |
| | |
| | |
| | |
| | |

## Psychoeducation Game Show Questions and Answers

1.  Draw the CBT triangle. (See diagram in chapter 1.)

    *     Earn an extra point if you draw the arrows correctly.

2.  True or **false**: People are just born with anxiety, and once they have it there is nothing they can do about it.

3.  What does the word "exposure" mean? (Exposure is when you do the thing that you fear.)

4.  **True** or false: Anxiety is something that is designed to protect you but can go off at the "wrong" time.

5.  True or **false**: The goal of treatment is to remove all anxiety so you never have to feel it again.

6.  Give two examples of exposures that could be helpful for someone who has a fear of roller coasters. (Watch videos of roller coasters, watch other people ride roller coasters, ride a small/large roller coaster)

7.  True or **false**: Medicatio n is the only helpful treatment for anxiety disorders.

For the next three questions, I'll give you choices, and you have to tell me which one is the best option:

8.  Here is a scenario: You wake up early and have anxiety about going to school. What should you do?

    A)   Go back to bed. It'll be easier tomorrow.

    B)   Get into an argument with Mom or Dad and hope they forget about taking you to school.

    C)   **Tell yourself that it may be hard to go, but you're up for the challenge and it will help your anxiety get better in the long run.**

9.  Which one of these is a goal of exposure therapy?

    A)   Totally freak you out and make you never want to come back to therapy.

    B)   **Work as teammates with your therapist to help you boss back your anxiety by slowly doing the things that make you nervous.**

    C)   Take away all your anxiety so you never feel it again.

10. Getting reassurance over and over again from friends, family, and your therapist is:

   A) A great solution to my problems

   B) Something that sometimes feels good in the moment but doesn't help my anxiety in the long run

   C) Something that we want to work to eliminate

   **D) Both B and C**

# PART II

# Getting Creative with Exposures for Anxiety and Related Disorders

# CHAPTER 5

# Specific Phobia

Part 1 provided an overview of exposure therapy as well as the general parameters for conducting exposures with younger clients and adults. Now, in part 2, we will discuss the various anxiety and related disorders for which exposure therapy is a large part of the treatment. We have provided creative exposures for you to use with your clients in order for them to be engaged, have fun (yes, it is possible), and target their core fears as best as possible. We begin with the specific phobias. In this chapter, we'll cover the diagnostic criteria as well as specific recommendations for you to keep in mind before diving into exposure.

## WHAT ARE SPECIFIC PHOBIAS?

Approximately 16% of adults and adolescents have a lifetime history of specific phobia (Kessler et al., 2012), making this the most common anxiety disorder. The *DSM-5* (APA, 2013) criteria for specific phobia include the following:

A.  The person has a marked, persistent, and excessive fear of a specific object or situation.

B.  Exposure to the feared object or situation almost always provokes an immediate anxiety response.

C.  The feared object or situation is avoided or endured with intense distress.

D.  The fear is out of proportion to the actual danger and the person's social or cultural context.

E.  The fear is persistent (e.g., six months or more).

F.  The fear or avoidance interferes significantly with the person's functioning or causes marked distress.

G.  The symptoms cannot be better explained by another mental disorder.

In order to meet diagnostic criteria for a specific phobia, the fearful reaction that clients experience when interacting with the feared situation must be intense or severe and must occur nearly every time the individual encounters or even anticipates coming into contact with the phobic situation.

## Types of Specific Phobias

While you can find exhaustive lists of specific phobias online (which many of you have likely seen) that range from ablutophobia (fear of washing or bathing) to zelophobia (fear of jealousy), in clinical practice, you're likely to encounter a more limited number. The specific phobias in the *DSM-5* are divided into five main categories:

**Natural Environment Type:** This category includes a fear of heights, thunder and lightning, and water.

**Blood-Injection-Injury Type:** This category includes fears of seeing blood, having blood draws or injections, and visiting the dentist. This is the only category that commonly includes fainting when presented with the feared situation.

**Animal Type:** This category includes fears of dogs, snakes, and insects.

**Situational Type:** This category includes fears of enclosed spaces or flying in airplanes.

**Other Types:** This category includes fears that do not neatly fit into one of the above-mentioned categories. Examples in this category can include fear of vomiting or choking, among others.

## Fear and Avoidance in Specific Phobia

Although people with specific phobias commonly describe their emotional reactions as fear, in some cases, the emotion experienced is disgust (Davey, 1993). Clients with phobias of some small animals (e.g., spiders) often describe the feared animal as disgusting rather than scary (de Jong, Andrea, & Muris, 1997). Similarly, clients with blood-injection-injury phobias may be particularly likely to describe their emotional reaction as disgust rather than fear (Sawchuk, Lohr, Tolin, Lee, & Kleinknecht, 2000). Disgust, thought to represent an evolutionary defense against contagion and disease (Rozin & Fallon, 1987), may be characterized by parasympathetic, rather than sympathetic, nervous system activation (Levenson, 1992). Some studies reported that clients high in *disgust sensitivity*, a trait-like predisposition to experiencing disgust, demonstrated less of an improvement in spider phobia symptoms following exposure therapy than did those low in disgust sensitivity (Merckelbach, de Jong, Arntz, & Schouten, 1993). Disgust during exposure usually does decrease over time; however, disgust reactions may decrease more slowly than do fear reactions (McKay, 2006; Olatunji, Smits, Connolly, Willems, & Lohr, 2007; Smits, Telch, & Randall, 2002), possibly indicating the need for more repetition of exposures (Vansteenwegen et al., 2007).

Specific phobias are usually characterized by a maladaptive pattern of avoidant behavior. For example, individuals with fears of storms might avoid going outside when the weather is bad. Those with blood-injection-injury fears might avoid having blood draws, injections, or trips to the doctor. Individuals with animal phobias might avoid going anywhere near the feared animal, which could include avoiding everyday activities like going for a walk, for fear of seeing someone else walking a dog. Those with flying phobias might avoid air travel altogether or might fly only with excessive use of alcohol or benzodiazepines (safety behaviors).

## Important Considerations in the Treatment of Specific Phobia

There is some conceptual overlap between specific phobia and other anxiety-related disorders. For example, a client with a specific phobia and one with agoraphobia might both be afraid of enclosed spaces or crowds. However, in the case of agoraphobia, it's important to note that the core fear is of panic-like or other embarrassing symptoms (e.g., throwing up, having diarrhea), rather than the situation itself. That is, an individual with agoraphobia is afraid not so much of an airplane crash (which might be the case in a specific phobia of flying), but rather of the possibility that he or she will have panic symptoms on an airplane and won't be able to escape the situation or get help. It's also noted that individuals with OCD might be afraid of blood; however, for those clients the core fear is usually that they will become contaminated, rather than fearing (or being disgusted by) the sight of blood (as would be the case in specific phobia).

# BEHAVIORAL TREATMENT FOR SPECIFIC PHOBIA

In the remainder of this chapter, we provide creative exposure ideas for the phobias you are most likely to encounter in your practice. However, it is our hope that once you are familiar with how to design and implement exposures, you will be able to successfully treat clients with any phobia who may walk through your door. We have chosen to list the exposure ideas from what many clients consider easiest to what many consider most challenging. However, it is important to note that every hierarchy you create with your client should be individualized. Some items that we list as a lower-level exposure may be at the top of your client's hierarchy of fears. Take the time to sit down with your client and rate these items from 0 to 100 (and generate your own ideas!).

For each type of phobia, we provide both "in-office" and "out-of-office" exposures. Note that all "out-of-office" exposures can be done with you and your client first, or you can assign any of the exposures for therapy homework.

## Natural Environment Phobias

This category includes a fear of weather events such as storms. Often it will be helpful to use imaginal exposure or virtual reality equipment to target many of these specific phobias—for example, to have a client experience a tornado—as they can be challenging to recreate in an office setting.

# Exposures for Fear of Storms

## In-Office Exposures: STORMS

- **Listen to audio clips of thunderstorms or tornados on your phone or computer.** Search online for "loud thunder clip" or "tornado sounds." You can have your client sit at your desk and type this into a search engine, or you can do it yourself with the client sitting next to you. You may want to begin with the volume low and then slowly increase it to make the exposure more challenging. You may find that one small piece of the clip is highly anxiety provoking, so you can keep playing that segment again and again for the client. Refrain from talking too much during the exposure as you do not want it to become a distraction for the client.

- **Watch video clips of storms (e.g., hurricane, thunderstorm, blizzard, tornado) or earthquakes on your computer.** Do an online search of "big storms" or "deadly storms." You can also consider having your client watch storm scenes from movies such as *Twister* or *The Perfect Storm*. Consider variables such as the volume on the video clips by starting it low and increasing it with future exposures. When this no longer is challenging, encourage your client to imagine being in the middle of the storm.

- **Write an imaginal exposure script of being in a feared storm.** Encourage the client to write a present-tense story about being in a terrible storm. Be specific! You can use the sample imaginal exposure script at the end of this chapter for inspiration.

- **Read online news stories of powerful storms.** Have the client search for and read scary stories about storms. Alternatively, you can read stories about deadly storms aloud to your client while he closes his eyes and pictures the story in his mind. It may be more challenging to have the client read the story aloud to you, so keep this in mind while creating the hierarchy.

- **Simulate thunder noises by drumming on a piece of sheet metal.** Once the client is comfortable with this, you can make these sounds outside of the window while he sits in the office alone, to be more realistic. You can also pair this with other exposures, such as when the client is reading his imaginal exposure script.

- **Use virtual reality (VR) equipment.** Some VR packages offer a "storm" package that can be used to help the client feel more immersed in the situation. Have the client wear the headset and/or headphones. If it is too challenging to wear both together, have the client do one at a time before combining them for the full storm experience.

## Out-of-Office Exposures: STORMS

- **Watch the weather channel.** If the client has been avoiding watching the news or weather for fear of thinking about or learning about upcoming storms, then it will be important to include exposures that allow the client to face this fear. Ask your client to keep the weather channel on while at home and also to watch episodes of shows that depict dangerous, and even deadly, storms.

- **Visit a science museum.** Sometimes science museums will have weather exhibits or simulators that replicate the experience of being in a storm, such as stepping inside of a wind machine, or hearing what it sounds like to be near a tornado or other kind of storm. Conduct an online search to see what exhibits may be present in your local museums.

- **Sit outside during a storm.** Encourage the client to sit on the porch or deck of his home when there is a storm (of course, if it is not hazardous to do so).

## Safety Behaviors to Eliminate: STORMS

Watch for signs of avoidance, such as your client going into the basement at any sign of a storm. Work with your client to eliminate this behavior, unless it is clearly necessary.

Watch also for excessive checking behavior, such as excessively checking the weather online to ensure that there are no storms coming. If these behaviors serve to lower the client's anxiety by reassuring him that no storm is coming, encourage the client to stop checking the weather. We are aware that earlier, we talked about watching the weather as an exposure. While it might seem like we're contradicting ourselves when we talk about eliminating this behavior, the distinction comes from what the client is currently doing. If the client is compulsively checking the weather as a means of reassuring himself, encourage the cessation of that behavior. Conversely, if the client is avoiding looking at the weather, encourage approach. The bottom line is that we want to reverse the client's current pattern of maladaptive behavior.

## Blood-Injection-Injury Phobias

Clients with blood-injection-injury (BII) phobias may fear going to the dentist or doctor, having injections, or having blood draws (or watching these happen to someone else). Some clients with BII phobias exhibit a vasovagal response, in which they faint or feel faint during or after exposure to the feared stimulus. In such cases, it's important to include an intervention to prevent fainting during exposure therapy. *Applied tension* (Kozak & Montgomery, 1981) is one such intervention. This method instructs clients to tense or "pump" their torso and thigh muscles repeatedly, which helps prevent pooling of the blood and increases blood flow to the brain. In BII phobia with vasovagal response, exposure with applied tension yields significantly better results than does exposure alone (Öst, Fellenius, & Sterner, 1991).

If your client is prone to fainting, be sure that you are conducting exposures in a manner and location that will not harm the client if he falls. Clients can engage in exposure exercises while sitting or reclining in a comfortable chair with arms, which not only improves blood flow to the brain, but also protects them from fall injuries. In case of actual fainting, the World Health Organization (2010) recommends having the client sit or lie in a reclined position, loosening any restrictive clothing, monitoring blood pressure if possible, giving the client something to drink, and offering reassurance. Recovery from fainting is usually rapid. An important psychological component of the intervention, in our opinion, is to "de-catastrophize" fainting so that the client does not view it as a failure experience or as the end of the world.

# Exposures for Fear of Blood, Injections, and Surgery

## In-Office Exposures: BLOOD, INJECTIONS, SURGERY

- **Look at online pictures of needles, blood, or people receiving injections.** You can start with having your client view cartoon pictures and increase to more intense pictures once the client has a sense of mastery over the easier ones. Have your client describe what he sees in the picture so that you can make sure the client is not engaging in subtle avoidance behaviors. For example, if the client is looking at a picture of a person receiving a blood draw, you can ask him to describe how the person looks (e.g., scared, relaxed), how big the needle is, if any blood is shown and how deep the color of the blood is, how the nurse looks taking the blood, and so on.

- **Use an alcohol swab.** Rub the client's arm with rubbing alcohol to simulate pre-injection procedures.

- **Use a tourniquet.** Tie a tourniquet around the client's arm to simulate pre-blood-draw procedures.

- **Look at and hold a syringe.** Keep the cap of a syringe on at first, then remove the cap, and then have the client practice removing the cap. Get comfortable playing with syringes!

- **Hold a syringe to the client's arm.** With the client's permission, place a syringe on his arm. This can first be done with the cap on, and then later you can do this exposure with the cap off of the syringe.

- **Use a blunt needle.** You can order blunt needles online and practice pressing them to the client's skin, as was done with the syringe example above.

- **Use imaginal exposure to feared consequences.** Work with your client to create an imaginal exposure script of fainting (or whatever the target feared outcome is) after getting an injection or a blood draw. Reference the sample imaginal exposure script at the end of the chapter.

- **Look at pictures of injections.** Conduct an online search with your client, which will provide you with a great range of pictures, from cartoons to photographs, ranging in degree of "bloodiness." Ask your client to rank these according to fear level. Keep a folder on your computer, or bookmark pages or pictures online, of those that were particularly challenging for your client so you can easily access them again for future exposures.

- **Watch instructional videos.** Conduct an online search with your client. Search terms such as "how to give an injection" or "how to draw blood" yield lots of clips. Sit with your client and watch these clips repeatedly. If the video is long, you can ask the client which part creates the most anxiety and then watch that portion of the clip repeatedly. You can also ask your client to describe exactly what is going on in the clip to make sure he is not engaging in cognitive avoidance by thinking about something else in order to feel less anxious.

- **Watch videos of blood draws.** Search online for "blood draw" or "venipuncture." Watch these videos with your client.

- **Watch videos of surgeries.** Search online for "thoracic surgery videos" or "plastic surgery videos." Have the client scan the video options and begin watching ones that are lower on the hierarchy and then move up to more challenging ones once the first ones are no longer anxiety producing. You can adjust the volume and the video screen size on your computer to titrate the dose of exposure—perhaps, for example, starting with a very small and quiet viewing, then gradually increasing the size and volume.

- **Watch scary movie scenes.** The movie *Saw II,* for example, has a clip with a person who jumps into a "needle pit." The movie *The Shining* has a scene in which blood comes gushing out of an elevator. The movie *Carrie* has a scene in which the title character gets covered with a bucket of blood. The movie *Reservoir Dogs* has multiple scenes of an injured character covered with blood. You and your client can find these movie clips online.

- **Test blood sugar.** You or your client can purchase an inexpensive kit at a drugstore or online to test his blood sugar by pricking his finger. You can later pair this exposure with the imaginal exposure script that the client created or with watching feared online clips of blood or injections.

## Out-of-Office Exposures: BLOOD, INJECTIONS, SURGERY

- **Sit for a blood draw without getting one done.** Have the client visit a phlebotomist or clinical laboratory (better yet, go with the client) and sit in the chair as if he were going to get an injection. Call ahead to the site and see if they will allow this.

- **Watch an injection.** If you, or the client's friend or family member, have an injection or a blood draw scheduled, encourage the client to come and watch.

- **Watch others donate blood.** Find out where the local blood drive is and then have the client visit the site (better yet, accompany the client to this) without any pressure to donate.

- **Go for acupuncture.** Schedule an appointment for acupuncture. During an acupuncture appointment, thin needles are placed into specific places on the body.

- **Get an injection.** Encourage the client to schedule a flu shot, blood draw, or other medically indicated injection. Accompany him if you can.

- **Donate blood.** Encourage the client to donate at a local blood drive.

# Exposures for Fear of the Dentist

## In-Office Exposures: FEAR OF THE DENTIST

- **View pictures of dental visits.** You can start by having your client look at cartoons of experiences at the dentist and increase this to more intense pictures once the client has a sense of mastery over the easier ones.

- **Listen to the sound of a dentist's drill.** Start by having your client listen to sounds of the drill alone and then add audio clips of a dentist drilling while someone is in pain or crying (search online for "dentist drill sounds"). Start with the volume low and steadily increase it to make the exposure more challenging. As the exposure becomes easier, encourage the client to imagine himself in the dentist's chair. Have your client repeatedly state, "This could be me."

- **Watch videos or clips online.** Search for "videos of dentist drilling cavity." Sit with your client while watching these.

- **Watch videos of having teeth pulled.** Search for "tooth extraction," and then later move to more challenging exposures such as "painful tooth extraction" or "tooth extraction gone wrong" and watch these together.

- **Use imaginal exposure to feared consequences.** Work with your client to create an imaginal exposure script of going to the dentist (or something bad occurring at the dentist). Once the client exhibits some degree of mastery over that task, have him read the script while an audio clip of drilling is playing in the background. There is an example imaginal exposure script provided at the end of the chapter.

## Out-of-Office Exposures: FEAR OF THE DENTIST

- **Drive to the dentist's office.** Drive with your client or ask him to go alone and sit in the parking lot without going into the office. Bring along the client's imaginal exposure script and ask him to read it while sitting in the parking lot of the dentist's office.

- **Sit in a dentist's waiting area.** With the dentist's permission, ask your client to sit in the dentist's waiting room without an appointment and observe what is occurring. He can also silently read the exposure script in the waiting room for a more challenging exposure.

- **Take a tour.** Have your client call ahead and ask to take a tour of the dentist's office.

- **Attend someone else's dental appointment.** Have your client go to a dental appointment with a friend or family member to watch what he has done (bonus points for viewing a cavity filling!).

- **Sit in a dentist's chair.** Have your client call ahead to the dentist's office and ask to sit in the chair and have the instruments (e.g., mirror) in his mouth.

- **Get a dental cleaning.** Ask your patient to have a dental cleaning with no cavities being worked on.

- **Complete dental work that has been delayed.** Have the client get a cavity filled or any other procedures done.

## Safety Behaviors to Eliminate: BLOOD, INJECTIONS, SURGERY; FEAR OF THE DENTIST

Many fearful clients take anxiolytic medications, such as benzodiazepines, before medical and dental procedures. Encourage the client to try these exposures without such medications, choosing instead to feel the fear and tolerate distress.

Watch for excessive reassurance-seeking. Asking once whether a procedure is likely to hurt is probably fairly normal. However, asking again and again for the purpose of feeling better is likely a safety behavior. Encourage the client to limit reassurance-seeking questions.

## Animal Phobias

Commonly seen fears within this category are of snakes, dogs, and bugs.

## Exposures for Fear of Snakes

### In-Office Exposures: SNAKES

- **Look at online pictures of snakes.** Start with having your client view cartoons and increase this to viewing more intense pictures (e.g., snakes shedding skin, snakes with large fangs, deadly snakes) once the client has a sense of mastery over the easier ones. Talk about what the client sees in each of these pictures.

- **Change the background/screensaver of a phone or computer.** Have the client put a picture of a snake as the background picture on his phone or on the desktop of his computer.

- **Talk about snakes.** Go back and forth with your client, coming up with words to describe snakes or their behavior (e.g., slithering, hissing, menacing, shedding skin).

- **Watch video clips of snakes.** Do an online search with your client for "videos of nice snakes" and then "videos of dangerous snakes" or "videos of snake biting someone." As is the case for other visually mediated phobias, you can change the dose of exposure by adjusting the size and volume of the video.

- **Create an imaginal exposure script.** Have your client include details in the story of coming into contact with a snake. Add what it feels like on the skin to hold the snake or to have it around one's neck. Reference the sample imaginal exposure script at the end of the chapter.

- **Wallpaper the home.** Print out pictures of various types of snakes, and give them to the client to hang up on the walls of his home to constantly be in contact with the feared stimulus.

- **Play with rubber snakes.** Order rubber snakes and put them on the office floor. You can also ask the client to hold the rubber snakes while going through other exposures, such as reading his imaginal exposure script aloud or watching videos of snakes.

## Out-of-Office Exposures: SNAKES

- **Get a new wallpaper for the phone or computer.** Have the client put a picture of a snake on the phone or computer lock screen or wallpaper.

- **Watch an entire movie about snakes.** For a homework assignment, have the client watch a documentary about snakes or a thriller movie such as *Snakes on a Plane*.

- **Visit a pet store.** Go with the client to the pet store if you can. Have the client take pictures of the snakes. The client can ask an employee to see the snake out of the cage (without holding it). Later on, ask the client to touch the snake or hold it. This may unfold over the course of several sessions.

- **Go on a snake hunt.** Go into the woods with your client on a "hunt" for snakes. Depending on where you go into the woods, it is fairly unlikely that you will come into contact with a snake, but the goal of the exposure is to have the client be willing to come into contact with one.

- **Have rubber snakes placed randomly throughout the home.** You can encourage your client to place rubber snakes randomly in his home to target the fear of being startled by these creepy crawly creatures. You can even ask the client's family members to be the ones in charge of placing these rubber snakes, with the client's permission. To make it more challenging, you can ask family members to randomly move them around the house throughout the week.

- **Visit a reptile house.** You can conduct an online search to find a nearby reptile house and go for a visit. You may be able to call ahead to ask if you can have a private showing of a snake and/or the opportunity to hold one.

# Exposures for Fear of Dogs

## In-Office Exposures: DOGS

- **Look at pictures of dogs.** Begin by having your client view pictures of cute puppies and work up to looking at pictures of bigger dogs, drooling dogs, or menacing-looking dogs. Have your client describe the details in the pictures.

- **Read scary stories about dogs.** Search online with your client for stories of dogs biting or attacking someone. Either read the stories aloud to your client or have your client read them aloud in the session.

- **Watch video clips of dogs.** Search online with your client for video clips of dogs doing cute things, and then work up to watching videos of barking dogs, dogs who jump, and a dog biting someone.

- **Create an imaginal exposure script.** Collaboratively create a story with your client of dogs attacking/biting/jumping around. Include details about how the dog smells, how it feels, what the barks sound like, and so on. Reference the sample imaginal exposure script at the end of this chapter.

- **Pet a dog.** If you have (or have access to) a dog, you can have the client touch the dog's face or mouth in session. Start with smaller dogs and work up to having the client be around larger dogs or jumpier dogs. You can begin with the dog on the leash and then consider having the dog off the leash when the client is more comfortable.

## Out-of-Office Exposures: DOGS

- **Visit a pet store.** Have your client go to a local pet store, where dogs are likely to be with some of the customers, either walking around the store or getting groomed. Once this becomes easier, the client can ask to hold or pet a dog in the pet store.

- **Go to a friend's or family member's home.** Ask your client to visit a friend or family member who has a dog and spend some time in the house without having the dog be put outside or in another room.

- **Give treats.** Have the client give a dog a treat from his hand.

- **Get licked by a dog.** Let the dog lick peanut butter off the client's hand.

- **Visit an animal shelter.** Have the client visit an animal shelter or volunteer at one.

- **Become a pet sitter.** Encourage the client to ask to pet sit a friend's or family member's dog for one night.

- **Visit a dog park.** Have your client stand outside the gate of a dog park and watch the dogs play. Accompany your client to the dog park, if possible. Once this becomes easier, have the client stand inside the gate of the dog park and watch the dogs play, or even throw balls for the dogs. Have the client move increasingly toward the center of the park and refrain from standing only in a spot where no dogs are playing or running around.

# Exposures for Fear of Bugs

## In-Office Exposures: BUGS

- **Look at pictures of bugs.** Start by looking at cartoon pictures of all different kinds of bugs (e.g., bees, cockroaches, flies, palmetto bugs), and then look at real pictures of these bugs online.

- **Watch video clips of bugs.** You can search online for insect videos, perhaps progressing to searches such as "people eating bugs" or "bug infestation."

- **Eat fake bugs.** Have the client eat chocolate or gummy candy in the shape of an insect (without actually eating an insect...that can come later!).

- **Make a bug purchase.** Have the client search online for, and then make an online purchase of, dehydrated bugs or tarantulas. Ask the client to bring them into session so that you can use them together for exposures.

- **Create a drawing.** Have the client draw a bug that is most terrifying to him. Ask the client to hang the picture up in a visible area of his home.

- **Create an imaginal exposure script of bugs.** Work with your client to create a detailed story of coming into contact with a bug. Make sure to add details to the story, such as how the bug feels crawling on the client and what noises (if any) the bug may make. Reference the sample imaginal exposure script at the end of the chapter.

- **Search for bugs.** Go on a "bug hunt" with your client and see who can spot the most bugs (and keep track!). Use the tracking sheet provided at the end of the chapter to play the bug game!

- **Look through a bug bag.** Have a bug bag on hand of dead bugs you've found. Have the client look at items in the bug bag without touching them.

- **Touch a bug.** Have the client reach into the bug bag and pull one out without looking at it.

- **Have a bug on the body.** Have the client put a dead bug on his lap. Work up to making the exposure more challenging by placing the bug on his bare skin.

- **Play a game of "catch" with a toy bug/spider or a real (dead) one.** Throw the bug back and forth with your client while saying words to describe the bug, such as "slimy" or "gross."

- **Catch a live bug.** Have your client catch a live bug and try to hold it or place it on his skin.

- **Eat real bugs.** Have the client eat a chocolate covered ant, grasshopper, cricket, or other insect that you can order online. Search online for "buy edible bugs."

## Out-of-Office Exposures: BUGS

- **Change the wallpaper on an electronic device.** Ask your client to put pictures of creepy, crawly bugs on either the lock screen of his phone or on the wallpaper of either his phone or computer. You can review this weekly in session and change it to more challenging photos each week.

- **Visit a science museum, "insect zoo," or museum of natural history.** Some museums will have exhibits on bugs, 3D movies about bugs, and sometimes an opportunity to touch bugs. There are several "insect zoos" and butterfly pavilions around the country as well, including at the Smithsonian. Check your local museums for more ideas to be used for exposure.

- **Visit a pet store.** Encourage your client to go to a pet store (with you, if possible) and look at all of the creepy crawly insects. Often, pet stores will sell crickets or roaches. The client can also purchase one to bring home to use for future exposures.

- **Create a client bug bag.** For homework, have the client go out and create his own bag of dead bugs and bring it to the next session.

- **Bring a bug home.** Allow the client to bring home one of the bugs that you both collected (or from your bug bag) and put it on the bedside table.

## Safety Behaviors to Eliminate: SNAKES; DOGS; BUGS

Many clients who engage in animal exposures tense their bodies, as if preparing to jump away from or otherwise avoid contact with the animal. Encourage a relaxed posture. It is also common for clients to hold their arms straight out when touching the feared animal, in order to keep the animal at arm's length from the body. Encourage closer contact.

Touching exposures often begin with just a fingertip. While this is acceptable as a first step, it can be a way for the client to minimize the exposure and feel safer. Encourage the client to use the whole hand (including the palm).

Discourage excessive reassurance-seeking. Asking once whether a snake, dog, or bug is likely to bite is a reasonable question, but it becomes a safety behavior when asked repeatedly. Encourage the client to limit reassurance-seeking questions.

## Situational Phobias

Situational phobias include excessive fears of specific situations such as heights, flying, and being in tight spaces.

## Exposures for Fear of Heights

### In-Office Exposures: HEIGHTS

- **Watch video clips.** Watch clips of people falling from high places. Conduct an online search for the movie *The Walk* to see a man tightrope across two high buildings.

- **Read stories.** Read stories of people who have been trapped high up on roller coasters or other structures. You can conduct an online search for "people who were stuck on roller coasters."

- **Use virtual reality equipment.** Use VR equipment to help the client feel as if he is high off the ground.

- **Create an imaginal exposure script.** With your client, create a detailed script of being high off the ground and include details of the client's feared outcome (e.g., falling, death).

- **Go up to the top of a building.** Take your client to a higher floor of the office building or parking garage, if possible. Have the client look down and repeatedly state, "I'm going to fall."

## Out-of-Office Exposures: HEIGHTS

- **Go to the top of a parking garage.** Ask your client to either walk or drive up to the top of a parking garage and stand close to the edge while looking down.

- **Climb a ladder.** Ask your client to practice going higher and higher up a ladder. You can even start out with a small step stool.

- **Visit an amusement park.** Have your client go to an amusement park and look up at the rides without any pressure to ride them.

- **Get in line.** Have your client get in line to go on a high waterslide or tall ride without following through and getting on the ride.

- **Ride the escalator.** Ask your client to ride an escalator in a shopping plaza while looking over the side. Ask your client to repeatedly think, *I could fall over the edge.*

- **Take an elevator.** Ask your client to ride in elevators in tall office buildings (this is often easier in a big city or in a hospital or business building). Glass elevators are also great options. Have the client start by just going up one floor and then work up to taking the elevator to the top floor. Standing with his forehead against the glass and looking down can intensify the sensation.

- **Cross a bridge.** Look up some nature walks or other places nearby where a client can visit a bridge to cross. Adjust the level of difficulty by changing up variables such as how old the bridge is, how high it is, and whether the client walks or drives on it.

- **Go on a ledge walk.** Depending on where you are located, there may be opportunities for your client to not only go to an elevated location but to also see directly beneath him due to a glass floor. Examples of such places in the United States include the Sears Tower and the Grand Canyon.

- **Go on a Ferris wheel or roller coaster.** Start by having your client ride smaller rides at the amusement park until he works up to riding on larger ones or ones that go higher and higher.

## Safety Behaviors to Eliminate: HEIGHTS

When the client is visiting a high place, he may keep far away from the edge as a safety behavior. Encourage the client to go as close to the edge as is safe. Also, when handrails are available in a high spot, some clients will grip them tightly, reducing their fear of falling. Encourage the client to let go of the handrail if it is safe to do so.

Some clients, in a high place, will avoid looking down. Sometimes this is because the client is trying to "forget" the height; in other cases, the client fears that looking down will cause vertigo, which then increases falling risk. Of course, true vertigo or other physical balance problems need to be considered carefully. However, in most cases, it is safe for the client to look down, and we recommend that he do so.

# Exposures for Fear of Flying

## In-Office Exposures: FLYING

- **Listen to sounds of a plane.** Do an online search with your client for airplane sounds. Allow this noise to play in the background while the client reads his imaginal exposure script.

- **Read stories.** Read stories with your client about scary or turbulent flights that ended well. Later the client can read stories about plane crashes. You can search online for "turbulent flights" or "scariest flight stories." He can read these stories aloud or you can read the stories to the client depending on how it is rated on the hierarchy.

- **Create an imaginal exposure script.** Work with your client to have him create a detailed script of a plane crashing or some other feared outcome (e.g., turbulence). Reference the imaginal exposure script at the end of the chapter.

- **Watch videos of flying.** There are many videos of flying available online that include take-off, landing, and what happens in flight. Some videos include smooth flights, while others have turbulence. Change these variables depending on the level of the client's anxiety and fear. After the client feels more comfortable with videos of turbulence, you can have him pair the videos with interoceptive exposures such as shaking or being jostled in a chair to simulate motion.

- **Use virtual reality equipment.** Have your client simulate the experience of being on a plane by using VR equipment.

- **Watch videos of plane crashes.** Several movies, including *Cast Away*, *The Grey*, and *Final Destination,* have clips of airplane crashes, from the passengers' point of view. You can find these clips online.

## Out-of-Office Exposures: FLYING

- **Drive to an airport.** Encourage you client to drive to the airport and sit in the parking lot without planning to take a flight.

- **Sit in the waiting area.** Have your client enter the airport, walk around, and sit in the ticketing area.

- **Take a ride.** Ask your client to schedule and attend a helicopter tour of a city.

- **Take a short flight.** Encourage your client to schedule a short flight. Often there are deals for flights that are less than $100.

- **Take a cross-country flight.** Have your client schedule a trip to a destination that he has previously avoided due to fear of flying.

- **Take an international flight.** Have your client take an international flight to an exciting destination.

- **Take a flying lesson.** Ask your client if he would be willing to sign up for a flying lesson.

## Safety Behaviors to Eliminate: FLYING

Alcohol and benzodiazepines are among the most commonly used safety behaviors when flying. Encourage the client to refrain from the use of sedating substances and to practice distress tolerance instead.

Some clients will "white-knuckle" the armrest on a plane, as if to keep the plane from crashing (we've even observed this phenomenon during VR exposure). Recommend a more relaxed grip.

A fearful flyer will often avoid looking out the window or looking around the plane (sometimes by keeping his face buried in a book or his eyes closed while listening to headphones). Encourage the client to look around and engage fully with the situation.

# Exposures for Fear of Tight Spaces

## In-Office Exposures: TIGHT SPACES

- **Look at pictures of enclosed spaces.** Search online with your client for "claustro-phobia pictures" and look through the items together.

- **Watch videos.** Conduct an online video search of people who have been trapped in caves or other small spaces and watch those together.

- **Say scary phrases.** Have your client close his eyes, picture a small space, and repeatedly say, "I'm trapped and can't get out."

- **Create a detailed imaginal exposure script.** Work with your client to create a detailed story about being trapped in a small space. Encourage your client to include lots of details in the story, such as the room or area feeling hot, becoming sweaty, and being unable to move around easily.

- **Have the client cover part of the face.** Have client wear a doctor's mask that covers the mouth and nose.

- **Place the client in a small area.** Ask the client to step into a small closet or small room. He can first do this alone and can then have others join him in a small room or closet to make it feel increasingly claustrophobic.

- **Say the worst fear aloud while in a small space.** Have the client go in a locked closet or room and repeatedly say, "I'm in a small space and can't get out."

- **Go into an elevator.** Step into an elevator with your client and stand inside it with the doors shut. Do not press a button to go to the next floor, so the elevator doesn't move and mimics the feeling of being stuck or trapped. This can be paired with the above exposure in which the client repeatedly states, "I'm in a small space and can't get out."

- **Wear a mask.** Have the client wear a Halloween-type mask that covers most of the face.

- **Be a burrito.** Ask the client to roll himself up into a rug, long blanket, or sheet until he is unable to move easily.

- **Get into a sleeping bag.** Get a sleeping bag or have the client bring one from home. Ask him to get into the sleeping bag head first.

- **Lock the client in a small closet, car trunk, or small room.** Yes, we know it's weird, and this is likely a high-level exposure that needs to be discussed and negotiated carefully within the context of a trusting therapeutic relationship. But for clients who are fearful of being trapped, it can be a useful experience. We recommend that at least at first, you remain right outside the door and talk the client through the exposure.

## Out-of-Office Exposures: TIGHT SPACES

- **Be in a small closet.** Have your client go into a small space or closet in his home in order to come in contact with that feared sensation of being closed in. To make it more challenging, the client can get into a sleeping bag in the closet or have a friend or family member wrap him up tightly in a blanket in the closet, and then shut the door.

- **Go into a mock MRI.** Have your client practice going into a mock MRI (some hospitals have these so that clients can acclimate to the scanner before having a real scan).

- **Ride a crowded subway.** Have your client ride on a crowded subway or bus at rush hour.

- **Go to a movie theater, concert, crowded church, or sporting event.** Have your client go to a movie theater or other seated area, and encourage him to sit in the middle of the aisle so that he is unable to get out easily.

- **Do an "escape room."** Escape rooms are adventure games in which players need to find clues and solve puzzles in order to escape a room before the clock runs out, which is usually an hour in length. Some of the rooms have locked doors, which will mimic the feeling of being in a small space and being unable to get out easily. In addition, in some of the more advanced rooms, players are handcuffed for a short period of time and need to find the key to "escape." These rooms often come with warnings that someone who is claustrophobic may not like the atmosphere and notify patrons in the beginning that they may leave the room at any time. Therefore, you and your client should explore these factors first before deciding which escape room to do.

## Safety Behaviors to Eliminate: TIGHT SPACES

Many clients with a fear of tight spaces will use deep breathing strategies to try to relax. This is not only a counterproductive safety behavior, but it also contributes to hyperventilation (which can be an exposure in its own right, if one is treating panic disorder). In most cases, we discourage the use of deep breathing as a coping strategy.

Some clients, when in a tight space, will avoid looking around or will even close their eyes, trying to trick their brain into forgetting where they are. Encourage the client to look around, recognize where he is, and tolerate the resulting distress.

## Other Types of Phobias

The "Other" category of phobias includes fears that do not neatly fit into one of the above-mentioned categories. Examples in this category can include fear of coming into contact with vomit (or vomiting) and fear of choking.

## Exposures for Fear of Vomit/Vomiting

### In-Office Exposures: VOMIT/VOMITING

- **Play a vomit word game.** Play a game where you and your client, and anyone else who is with you during the exposure (e.g., confederate, client's parent), has to alternate saying words that either describe vomit or are synonyms for the word vomit. Here are a few suggestions: chunky, beefy, bile, oozing, wet, barf, blow chunks, puke, projectile vomit, splattering, thick, juicy, heave, hurl, regurgitate, spew.

- **Listen to sounds of vomiting.** Search online for audio files of "vomit sounds." You can start the volume low and slowly increase it to make the exposure more challenging. You can later ask your client to try to mimic the sounds that he hears in the videos.

- **Look at pictures of people vomiting.** You can start with having the client look at cartoon characters vomiting and then advance to real people getting sick. The website http://www.ratemyvomit.com has literally thousands of photographs of people throwing up.

- **Play the jelly bean game with your client (see additional page for directions).** Have your client eat gross-flavored jelly beans (such as vomit, skunk, or spoiled milk) to target feeling sick or as if he could vomit. You can play this game as a way to make the exposure more fun—younger clients especially love it. You will need to purchase BeanBoozled Jelly Beans, which are made by Jelly Belly. There are some packs of jelly beans you can purchase that come with a spinner. For these, the client will have to eat the jelly bean the spinner lands on. There are other jelly beans that come in a canister that pushes one jelly bean to the top, so you never know which one will be the one you get.

- **Eat vomit-flavored jelly beans.** Have your client eat vomit-flavored jelly beans while watching video clips of people vomiting. You can also search for "BeanBoozled challenge" to view clips of people gagging or even vomiting while eating the jelly beans.

- **Make fake vomit.** Make a concoction with your client that looks like vomit.

  Here's a recipe for fake vomit:[*]

  > 2 cups cottage cheese
  >
  > ¼ cup sour cream
  >
  > 1 package onion soup mix
  >
  > 1 small carrot (diced)
  >
  > 4 drops or more of yellow food coloring

  Here's another fake vomit recipe:

  > 1 can beef and barley soup
  >
  > 1 can cream of mushroom soup
  >
  > ½ cup sweet relish
  >
  > ½ cup vinegar

- **Fake vomit into toilet.** Take the created vomit concoction and have the client stand over the toilet and mimic sounds of heaving while plopping some of the mixture into the toilet. Be sure to encourage your client during this time by saying things like "Whoa, you got a lot up that time!"

- **Use a tongue depressor.** Ask your client to put a straw or tongue depressor in his mouth to get the gag reflex going. The point of this exercise is not to induce vomiting, but rather to feel the sensations of gagging.

- **Watch a video clip of someone vomiting.** Watch online videos together of people vomiting. You can begin with cartoon characters vomiting and then advance to real people vomiting. You can find seemingly endless examples online. Ideas from cartoons include a *Family Guy* episode where there is an ipecac drinking contest (Season 4, episode 8). Ideas from popular movies include *Pitch Perfect,* in which a character vomits on stage while performing, *Monty Python's The Meaning of Life,* which has a cartoonish scene of repeated vomiting, and *Stand By Me,* which contains a rather preposterous scene of an entire crowd of people vomiting.

- **Consume food or drink that was previously avoided due to fear.** Rank order a list of foods that your client avoids due to fear of vomiting, and systematically work up the hierarchy, allowing him to try each item repeatedly until the anxiety comes down. Many times, clients are wary of dairy items or raw items such as sushi. You can ask your client to bring in a feared item (e.g., yogurt), and then after the exposure, tell him you will keep it in your refrigerator until the next session for him to taste (we wouldn't do this with sushi, though). This is particularly effective since the client can't check it, and the item will already have been opened and "exposed" to other things in the refrigerator that the client may fear could make him sick.

---

[*]    We'd like to thank our colleague Mary Alvord for passing these recipes along.

## Out-of-Office Exposures: VOMIT/VOMITING

- **Wallpaper the home with pictures of vomit.** Print out cartoons of vomit or characters vomiting and have your client "wallpaper" his house (or bedroom) with the pictures to constantly be exposed to the feared stimulus. Once this becomes easier, you can have the client hang more graphic pictures of vomiting around the house or a room in the house.

- **Get a new wallpaper for the phone or computer.** Have the client put a picture of a cartoon or real person vomiting on the phone or computer lock screen or wallpaper.

- **Go to a party.** Ask your college-aged students to attend college parties as there may be others there who are intoxicated and throwing up.

- **Go to a restaurant.** Ask your client to go to a restaurant and eat previously avoided food, such as sushi or a hamburger/steak that is cooked at a medium or a medium-rare temperature.

- **Visit a hospital.** Have your client walk around a hospital, where he could come into contact with a person who is sick who poses a risk of contamination and subsequent vomiting.

- **Visit a theme park.** Encourage your client to ride on a roller coaster or other ride that could lead to motion sickness (and therefore a risk of vomiting).

## Safety Behaviors to Eliminate: VOMIT/VOMITING

Many clients will take steps to avoid vomiting, including taking deep or slow calming breaths, using (or carrying) antiemetic medication, chewing gum, or carrying a water bottle. Encourage the client to drop these behaviors during exposure and to practice fear tolerance instead. Other clients will engage in behaviors designed to mitigate the effects of vomiting, such as carrying bags, being near a trash can, or staying near an exit. Encourage the elimination of these behaviors.

# Exposures for Fear of Choking

## In-Office Exposures: CHOKING

- **Listen to an audio recording of people choking.** Do an online search for "choking noises" with your client.

- **Look at pictures of people choking.** Start by searching online for cartoons of people choking, and then increase the intensity to looking at pictures of real people choking.

- **Watch video or movie clips of people choking.** Watch a clip from the movie *Mrs. Doubtfire* in which the lead character chokes while eating at a restaurant. You can also search online for "real choking videos" to see clips of people choking and receiving the Heimlich maneuver.

- **Read online stories about people choking.** Search online for stories of people who have choked on food items.

- **Practice rapid swallowing.** Have your client target the feared sensation of choking by rapidly swallowing with nothing in his mouth. This can mimic the sensation of the throat becoming tense.

- **Imaginal exposure to choking.** Have the client imagine chewing and swallowing food that is difficult to swallow, like a large piece of chewy steak. Describe what it would feel like getting stuck in the throat, as well as the feared consequence (e.g., getting the Heimlich maneuver, trying to do the Heimlich over the side of a chair or table while alone, or dying).

- **Combine viewing videos of choking with eating.** In session with your client, watch videos of choking while your client eats a snack of a feared food item.

- **Pretend to choke.** Have the client grab his throat to make the sign that he is choking and make gasping noises.

- **Hold a non-food item in the mouth.** Have your client place a small item in the front of his mouth (e.g., a water bottle cap, a small plastic toy that has a hazardous warning to children under three on it).

- **Eat foods that tend to make you want to reach for a drink.** Have your client eat a spoonful of peanut butter without drinking anything to help it get down.

- **Swallow pills.** Have the client swallow an over-the-counter medication (e.g., vitamin pill, Tylenol) with water. Later, make this more challenging by having the client swallow a pill without any fluid.

- **Work through a food hierarchy.** Systematically introduce any specific foods (e.g., mozzarella sticks, steak sandwich, hot dogs, grapes) that the client has been avoiding. Start with a bite and gradually increase the amount he eats in session.

## Out-of-Office Exposures: CHOKING

- **Swallow food items at home.** Have the client practice swallowing small food items (e.g., tic tacs) at home when in the company of others, then when alone.

- **Watch video clips of choking.** Have the client view these clips while eating at home alone.

- **Eat feared food items while home alone.** Have the client work through a food fear hierarchy that you and he created in session. Consider including "sharp" foods like tortilla chips as they can scrape the side of the esophagus and feel uncomfortable if the piece was too big.

- **Go out to restaurants.** Ask the client to go to a restaurant by himself and eat items that are higher up on the food fear hierarchy.

## Safety Behaviors to Eliminate: CHOKING

Eating in the presence of other people is a common safety behavior for clients with fears of choking (presumably because the other person can administer first aid or call 911 in case of choking). Encourage the client to practice eating alone.

Many clients with fear of choking severely limit what they eat, often sticking to liquids or soft foods. Encourage the gradual incorporation of more challenging foods. Some clients with choking fears will carry a water bottle in case of food getting "stuck." Encourage them to leave the water bottle at home. Finally, some clients who fear choking will overchew food to minimize the perceived risk of choking. Encourage a normal amount of chewing.

# CONCLUSIONS

Specific phobias can be of the natural environment (e.g., storms); blood, injections, or injuries; animals (e.g., dogs, snakes, insects); specific situations (e.g., enclosed spaces, flying); or other situations or activities including vomiting or choking. Specific phobias are best addressed using in vivo exposure to the feared situation or activity, though in some cases imaginal or virtual reality exposure can be used. As with all fears, be vigilant for the presence of safety behaviors and strive to eliminate them wherever possible.

In the next chapter, we will review diagnostic criteria for panic disorder and agoraphobia and provide both interoceptive and in vivo exposure ideas for addressing these conditions.

# CHAPTER RESOURCES

**Reminder:** These resources are also available to download and print from http://www.newharbinger.com/43737.

## Example Imaginal Exposure Script—*Storms*

*An ominous green haze covers the sky as the warning alarms in my town begin to sound. There was not supposed to be a storm today. There is nowhere to run or hide, as a tornado can change its path at any moment. The alert on my phone comes through, which increases my heart rate. The tornado is approaching. I must brace myself immediately. I'm all alone and the most terrified I have ever been in my life. I frantically search for the safest part in my home where I will least likely be hit by falling debris. The lights in my home flicker and then suddenly go out. I am in complete darkness. I hear the pounding rain outside. All of a sudden I hear a loud noise in the distance that sounds as if it is getting closer. It is as if a freight train is coming straight for my home. I hide myself fully under a mattress and close my eyes as I hear the shingles of my roof being ripped off of my home. Things are falling all around me. I feel the outside air and know I am exposed and no longer safe in my own home. This is it. This is how it all ends.*

## Example Imaginal Exposure Script—*Blood*

*I open the door to the phlebotomist's office to get my blood drawn and before even checking in for the appointment I am filled with fear. With no time to even consider leaving, I hear my name being called. I am seated in a large chair where many before me have had their blood taken. As soon as that thought crosses my mind, I try to push it away. I place my arm on the chair, palm side facing up. I can barely get my eyes to focus while the technician grabs a tourniquet and tightens it around my upper arm. I am given a squishy ball to hold and asked to clench my fist to help find a good vein. Sweat beads up on my forehead and my free arm grabs the arm of the chair, bracing for the worst. I see the needle lying on the table next to a stack of test tubes. Are those all for me to fill? What if I faint? As if in slow motion, the technician takes a cotton ball and alcohol to wipe down the area of my arm that the needle will stab. I hear the cap of the needle fall to the metal table as the tip of the long, silver needle meets my skin. I feel the sting of the needle and think this must be over soon, but the needle stays in and more and more vials of blood are collected. I try to focus my eyes on the notices taped on the concrete wall of the sterile room, but my eyes won't adjust. The room starts to spin around me and as I begin to tell the technician I feel sick, I feel my body begin to go limp.*

## Example Imaginal Exposure Script—*Dentist*

*I arrive at the dentist's office and walk inside. It smells sterile and uninviting. I feel a shiver run through my body. I can hear the drill in the background and know that it will soon be my turn. I sit in the office in an uncomfortable chair looking around at all the mini-size freebies of mouthwash, floss, and toothpaste. My hands are shaky and my mouth dry. The dental hygienist calls my name and brings me back into the present moment. I follow her to the room to have X-rays taken. Minutes later the dentist comes in and says, "You're going to have to have that cavity filled." He asks me to open my mouth and try to relax. How can I relax? I grip the sides of the chair and brace for impact. He's trying to relax me by talking about summer vacation plans, but I can't be distracted. I feel the sting of the Novocain needle. What if it won't be enough? What if I feel the drill? What if I need to run out of here crying? As soon as I am numbed, the dentist grabs the drill and turns it on. The high-pitched sound makes me cringe. Hot tears start to fall down my face. I'm panicking. This is my worst fear. I brace myself as I hear the drill touch my tooth. I feel it! I feel it! I don't have enough Novocain. I knew this would happen. I raise my hand to gesture for him to stop. He does. He tells me he will need to give me another shot of Novocain before we can move forward. He does just that. He drills and drills and drills. The whirling sound echoes in my ears. Will this ever end?*

## Example Imaginal Exposure Script—*Snakes*

*I am sitting outside relaxing on a warm, sunny day when I feel a cold and slimy sensation touch the back of my ankle. I look down and see a big ugly black and red snake. I jump back, knocking my glass of iced tea off the table and onto the floor. The snake is frightened and gets into a menacing stance as if poised to strike. The snake is about eighteen inches long and has a slender but muscular body. I can't help but notice the pink tongue that flashes in and out of its mouth, and every few seconds I see a piece of its yellowish fang. I feel a flash of panic run through my entire body as I have the urge to run but am too scared it will chase me—or even worse. I stand frozen in my spot, scanning my mind for escape options. I reach for a stick in hopes that I can scare it off when I see movement out of the corner of my eye. There must be at least three more snakes! They are so close to each other that I cannot see where one ends and the other begins. I hear a hissing sound as the scaly and menacing creatures slither toward me. I am paralyzed with fear.*

## Example Imaginal Exposure Script—*Dogs*

*I decide to take a quick walk on my lunch break, and I see a man across the street walking his massive dog. The dog appears to be a mixed breed of some sort—maybe German shepherd and Rottweiler. I can immediately tell it is not friendly. I start moving faster as I feel my fear increasing. I hear the owner yell from across the street, "No! No! Stay!" The owner has completely lost control of the dog, which begins thrashing around and wiggles its neck out from the spiky collar. The dog's leash and collar are now lying on the ground by the owner. In an instant, the dog takes off across the street with his eyes glued to me. I am his target. The dog doesn't slow as he approaches me and I am suddenly knocked to the pavement. He snarls at me as if I am his worst enemy. His big white teeth clench down on my right forearm as I struggle to hit him with my other hand. There is blood everywhere. The dog's owner runs toward us and keeps calling the dog's name and telling him "No!" but he is unable to grab the dog without his leash or collar. There is nothing I can do. I am helpless.*

## Example Imaginal Exposure Script—*Bugs*

*I'm lying in my bed, with my eyes closed, and I feel a tingling sensation on my hand. I open my eyes, and it's a giant, hairy bug, looking right at me. I feel paralyzed with fear. I can feel each of its legs on my skin as it crawls over my hand. I don't want to look at it, but I'm afraid to look away. My heart is racing and I feel like I can't breathe. Slowly I look down toward my feet and I see that there are dozens, maybe hundreds, of bugs all over me! They're crawling and slithering over my legs, my stomach, and my chest. My skin feels like it's crawling. I'm terrified but I can't move; I can't just get up and shake the bugs off. They're going to stay on me. I look back to the big bug on my hand and see that it's now crawling up my arm, making its way toward my face. All I can feel are the bugs all over my skin and my own heart pounding out of my chest. I can hear the bugs clicking and hissing as they crawl on me. The big bug has made its way up to my face now. I shut my eyes and close my mouth tightly to prevent the bug from getting in, but it's headed toward my ear. I think it's going to crawl into my ear and possibly lay eggs in there. As the bug crawls into my ear, the pack of bugs keep making their way up my body until they are covering my face. I'm trying not to breathe, but I can feel them making their way into my nostrils and my mouth. I want to scream but I can't because there are bugs all over my mouth.*

## Example Imaginal Exposure Script—*Flying*

*I'm on the plane and I'm already feeling nervous. What if something happens to the plane? My heart is racing and I wish we would just land already. The pilot comes on the intercom, and I think I hear him say something about turbulence, but I can't hear him very clearly because of all of the people talking. When we hit the first bump, I immediately grip my armrests. What's happening? My heart is really pounding now and I'm feeling very scared. Another bump and now the flight attendant hurries back to her seat and buckles in. I'm getting more and more scared, feeling like my chest is going to explode. Now the bumps are coming more rapidly and more strongly. It feels like we're hitting things in the air, the way the plane is lurching. The people on board have become quiet and all I can hear now is the sound of the engines. They sound like they're whining, like something's wrong with them. I look around, panicked, and see that other people on the plane have fearful faces. One woman is crying. Another man looks like he's praying. The plane does a sudden drop and everyone on board screams. I'm panicking but there's nothing I can do; I'm strapped in a seat 30,000 feet in the air. Now the plane drops down again and keeps going. The flight attendant yells out, "Assume crash position!" Everyone on the plane is screaming now. I put my head between my legs and I know I'm about to die as we plummet down.*

## Example Imaginal Exposure Script—*Choking*

*I'm at home alone eating a sandwich. As I swallow, I feel something is stuck in my throat. I go to get a glass of water from the kitchen sink, but no water comes out of the tap. I feel like I can't breathe. I'm getting really scared and I realize that I'm choking. In a panic, I open the refrigerator door looking for something to drink but there's nothing in there. My throat is full and I can't swallow, breathe, or talk. I try pushing on my stomach but that doesn't help. My face is getting red, and it feels like there's a pressure coming from behind my eyes. I'm terrified and I think that I'm choking to death. There's no one home to help me. Frantically I look for my phone to call 911 but I can't find it. The room seems to be spinning as I'm running out of air. I drop to my knees, clutching at my throat. I try to scream but no sound comes out. As I slide to the floor I realize I'm dying.*

## Rules of the Jelly Bean Game

Your therapist has a mixture of jelly beans for you to try. Some are delicious, like juicy pear, and some are…not so delicious, like booger.

**Goal of the game:** Earn as many points as you can to cash them in for a reward (decide this reward with your therapist/parent/spouse). You will find the points for each pairing below. Since each gross jelly bean has a yummy counterpart, you will earn the same amount of points if it turns out to be a "good" jelly bean or a "bad" one. You get the points for taking a risk and trying it!

**Additional directions:** In order to get the points for choosing one of the jelly beans below, you must chew the bean at least three times. No partial points will be awarded. At any time in the game, you can "steal" a barf jelly bean for an additional 5 points!

**We dare you not to vomit!**

Jelly Bean Pairs

- Dead Fish—Strawberry Banana Smoothie (1 point)
- Spoiled Milk—Coconut (1 point)
- Stinky Socks—Tutti-Frutti (1 point)
- Lawn Clippings—Lime (1 point)
- Toothpaste—Berry Blue (1 point)
- Rotten Egg—Buttered Popcorn (2 points)
- Canned Dog Food—Chocolate Pudding (2 points)
- Booger—Juicy Pear (2 points)
- Caramel Corn—Moldy Cheese (2 points)
- Barf—Peach (3 points)

## Let's Go on a Bug Hunt!

**Goal:** Find as many bugs as you can. Play as a team or against one another to see who can find the most bugs! Search online for any bugs you do not know the name of so that you can include the information below.

| Bug Type | Bug's Color | Bug's Length | Other Characteristics (e.g., flying, noises it makes) |
|---|---|---|---|
|  |  |  |  |
|  |  |  |  |
|  |  |  |  |
|  |  |  |  |
|  |  |  |  |
|  |  |  |  |
|  |  |  |  |

# CHAPTER 6

# Panic Disorder and Agoraphobia

In this chapter, we will discuss exposure therapy for panic disorder and agoraphobia. After reviewing the criteria of these disorders and important treatment considerations, we will provide exposure ideas for facing fears of physiological sensations by using interoceptive exposures. We will also include creative in vivo exposure ideas to target the fear of confined spaces or feeling trapped, crowded areas, and open spaces as is seen in clients with agoraphobia. Finally, we will provide ideas for imaginal exposure exercises.

## WHAT IS PANIC DISORDER?

Nearly 7% of adults in the United States have a lifetime history of panic disorder, and nearly 4% have a lifetime history of agoraphobia (Kessler et al., 2012). Agoraphobia frequently co-occurs with panic disorder (Kessler et al., 2006); hence, we combine them in this chapter.

According to the *DSM-5* (APA, 2013), the criteria for panic disorder are:

A. Having four or more of the following symptoms during an unexpected panic attack (defined as "an abrupt surge of intense fear or intense discomfort that reaches a peak within minutes" [p. 208]):

1. Palpitations, pounding heart, or accelerated heart rate

2. Sweating

3. Trembling or shaking

4. Feeling of shortness of breath or of being smothered

5. A feeling of choking

6. Chest pain or discomfort

7. Nausea or stomach distress

8. Feeling dizzy, unsteady, lightheaded, or faint

9. Chills or hot flashes

10. Numbness or tingling sensations which are usually in the hands, feet, or face (paresthesias)

11. Feelings of unreality (derealization) or being detached from the self (depersonalization)

12. Fear of losing control or going crazy

13. Fear of dying

B. At least one of the attacks has been followed by at least a month of worry about having a future panic attack or the potential consequences of having panic attacks, such as having a heart attack, or some change in behavior as an attempt to avoid having another panic attack.

C. The symptoms are not better accounted for by a medical condition, medication use, or substance use.

D. The disturbance must not be better explained by another mental health disorder. For example, panic attacks only occurring in response to feared social situations (e.g., giving a speech, making small talk) would be better accounted for by a diagnosis of social anxiety disorder.

## Panic Attacks vs. Panic Disorder

Panic attacks are a relatively normal phenomenon that many of us will experience in our lifetime. It is important to remember that having a panic attack is not the same thing as having panic disorder. Panic attacks are necessary, but not sufficient, for the diagnosis of panic disorder. A panic attack is a brief, intense episode of anxiety that can be triggered by something in particular, such as seeing a spider in the case of specific phobia, or can occur out of the blue, for no apparent reason at all, in unexpected situations.

Individuals with panic disorder, unlike those with panic attacks due to other anxiety-related disorders, experience multiple unexpected panic attacks. They then worry about when and where the next attack might occur. Due to the fear of future attacks, individuals with panic disorder may start avoiding situations in which they think there is a chance of having a panic attack. For example, an individual may have had her first panic attack while at the grocery store. The person then stops going to the grocery store, or she goes during times when there are not many people shopping (e.g., late at night or first thing in the morning). The individual's fear of the grocery store may begin to generalize to the point where she may then start avoiding other stores, such as shopping malls, banks, coffee shops, and so on. This is how agoraphobia (see below) can develop.

## Is Panic Dangerous?

Despite the fact that panic attacks are extremely uncomfortable, it is important for the client (and the therapist) to recognize that they are not dangerous. People with panic disorder may present to the emergency room thinking that they are having a heart attack or some other serious medical emergency. This is often because the symptoms of panic, such as heart racing or pounding, lightheadedness, and tingling sensations, are misinterpreted as catastrophic in nature (i.e., that they are symptoms of a heart attack). The goal of exposure treatment is not to escape the uncomfortable physiological sensations and to make sure they never occur again, but rather to face them, experience them, and help the client to recognize that they are harmless.

# WHAT IS AGORAPHOBIA?

The criteria for agoraphobia listed in the *DSM-5* (APA, 2013) are:

A. Significant fear of at least two of the following situations:

1. Using public transportation, such as planes, trains, subways, or buses

2. Being in open spaces, such as parking lots or bridges

3. Being in enclosed spaces, such as shops or theaters

4. Standing in line or being in a crowd

5. Being outside of the home alone

B. The individual avoids the above situations due to fear that escape may be challenging and/or help might not be readily available should panic-like or embarrassing symptoms arise, such as incontinence or vomiting.

C. These situations must almost always provoke fear or anxiety.

D. The situations are either actively avoided or endured with intense anxiety or discomfort and may require the presence of a companion, such as a parent or spouse.

E. Fear or anxiety is out of proportion to actual threat or danger.

F. Fear, anxiety, or avoidance is persistent and lasts six months or more.

G. Fear, anxiety, or avoidance must cause significant distress or interference in important areas of functioning.

H. Should a medical condition be present (e.g., irritable bowel syndrome, Parkinson's disease), the fear, anxiety, or avoidance must be excessive.

I. Fear, anxiety, or avoidance is not better accounted for by another psychiatric disorder, such as a specific phobia or social anxiety disorder.

# PANIC DISORDER AND AGORAPHOBIA: CLINICAL CONSIDERATIONS

In this section, we will discuss issues pertinent to both panic disorder and agoraphobia, either combined (most common) or in isolation.

## Fear and Avoidance in Panic Disorder and Agoraphobia

It is easy to miss the core fear in panic disorder and agoraphobia. Individuals with these disorders commonly come to treatment describing a fear of external stimuli—for example, clients describe a fear of driving in traffic, a fear of crowded shopping malls, and so on. And while it is certainly true that these situations are often feared and avoided, they are not the core fear. At their heart, panic disorder and agoraphobia represent a *fear of fear* (Goldstein & Chambless, 1978). Individuals with panic disorder and agoraphobia are fundamentally afraid of their own physiological fear reactions, and what they think those reactions signify. Clients may believe, for example, that:

- Racing heart means I am going to have a heart attack.

- Dizziness means I am going to pass out.

- Upset stomach means I am going to throw up.

- Derealization means I am going crazy.

- Various other signs or symptoms of the "fight-flight-freeze" response mean I am going to panic and lose control of myself.

When we conceptualize panic and agoraphobia as a fear of fear, these disorders become much easier to understand. Panic attacks, though they may be unexpected, do not come from nowhere. Rather, the cycle (see our CBT triangle figure in chapter 1) begins with an uncomfortable but benign physiological sensation, such as elevated heart rate or butterflies in the stomach. The person then engages in distorted patterns of thinking such as *probability overestimation* (e.g., *I am going to have a heart attack*) or *catastrophizing* (e.g., *If I experience a panic attack, it means I will run amok like a crazy person and have to be hospitalized*). These cognitive distortions, in turn, lead the person to feel even more fearful, and around and around it goes, often culminating in a panic attack (Clark, 1986).

The person's behavioral response to this "fear of fear" pattern, not surprisingly, is often one of avoidance. People with agoraphobia will often avoid situations in which escape would be difficult or help would not be immediately available in case of a panic attack or panic-like symptoms. So, for example, a client who fears having a panic attack might avoid going to crowded places (such as a shopping mall), driving in heavy traffic, or being far away from home, in case she feels panicky and won't be able to escape easily or get help from others.

The avoidance in panic and agoraphobia can also be of internal stimuli (i.e., avoidance of feelings and physiological sensations). Because of their fear of fear, many clients with panic and agoraphobia will avoid activities that stimulate physiological arousal. This can include avoidance of exercise, avoidance of scary movies, avoidance of caffeine, avoidance of sex, and avoidance of strong emotions. In each case, the individual is trying to keep her physiological arousal level low in the hopes that this will reduce or eliminate the perceived risk of disastrous consequences.

Finally, we should note that individuals with panic and agoraphobia very frequently use a variety of safety behaviors that, while soothing, can be counterproductive. Clients may be reluctant to leave home without a bottle of benzodiazepines, a cell phone, a bottle of water, or some other "crutch." In many cases, that "crutch" is another person; for example, a client might be willing to go to the mall only in the presence of her spouse because of the mistaken belief that the spouse will "rescue" her from the situation in the event of a panic attack or panic-like symptoms.

## Important Considerations in the Treatment of Panic Disorder and Agoraphobia

The avoidant behavior in agoraphobia can resemble that of specific phobia (see chapter 5). For example, clients with either condition might avoid certain situations such as flying in an airplane. The critical difference is what is feared. The client with a specific (flying) phobia generally fears that the plane is going to crash, whereas the client with agoraphobia fears that she will have a panic attack or panic-like symptoms and will not be able to escape while on the plane or will become embarrassed. This distinction has important implications that go beyond the diagnostic label. When a client is afraid of plane crashes, we might be well advised to use in vivo exposure to air travel when possible, or perhaps imaginal exposure or VRET that relates specifically to being on an airplane. However, when a client is afraid of fear, panic, and panic-like symptoms, it is critical to also include interoceptive exposure so that you can expose the client to the fearful sensations themselves.

## Involving a Safety Person in Treatment

As we have mentioned, agoraphobia is a fear of being trapped or stuck in a place where escape may not be easy or help might not be available, and the individual fears her own fearful emotions and bodily sensations. For example, the client may fear becoming nauseated and throwing up while in a crowded place where she may not be able to escape easily, such as a packed movie theater, thus becoming embarrassed. Sometimes, an individual with such a concern may be less anxious (and more willing to enter feared situations) in the presence of a "safety person." A safety person might include a spouse, parent, friend, or other trusted companion. This person might accompany the client in only very high stress situations, such as flying or going long distances away from home, or the relationship can evolve to the point where the client goes very few places (or no places at all) without the safety person.

This safety behavior of bringing a trusted companion with the client is an important target for treatment, as you will want to work with your client to have her gain the confidence to enter feared situations alone. Therefore, we recommend including the safety person in the client's treatment, with the client's permission. You may ask your client to bring her safety person to early sessions to join in exposures with the goal of eventually having the client do exposures on her own, without being accompanied by the safety person. The safety person will also benefit from psychoeducation to understand the role of avoidance and safety behaviors, and how you are working with your client to systematically eliminate the avoidance behaviors.

# BEHAVIORAL TREATMENT FOR PANIC DISORDER AND AGORAPHOBIA

Although panic disorder can occur with or without agoraphobia, these two disorders frequently co-occur (Grant et al., 2006; Kessler et al., 2006) and have a common core mechanism (fear of fear). Thus, we have combined our discussion of exposures for these two overlapping disorders in this chapter. We have organized this chapter according to the three types of exposure that we discussed in chapter 3:

1.  Interoceptive exposures

2.  In vivo exposures

3.  Imaginal exposures

## Interoceptive Exposures

Chapter 3 will be a handy resource when working with your clients with panic and/or agoraphobia as it includes additional information on how to do interoceptive exposures, which are a major part of the treatment for panic and agoraphobia. Chapter 3 also includes worksheets that will be useful to you, so we suggest reviewing that section. Some clinicians might be uncomfortable doing and prescribing interoceptive exposures with clients who have panic disorder. After all, as clinicians, we want our clients to feel *better*, and interoceptive exposures can definitely make them feel *worse* (at least in the short term), which is normal when conducting any kind of exposure. However, the importance of interoceptive exposure in panic and agoraphobia cannot be overstated: we consider it to be *the* central feature of CBT for these conditions.

This is a time when that sneaky exposophobia may begin telling you that interoceptive exposure is a risky intervention that should be avoided. First, don't avoid. Second, go ahead and do some practicing on your own! We recommend practicing doing all of the interoceptive exposures first by yourself before asking your clients to do them. This way you'll get the hang of them, realize they are not as bad as you might imagine, and feel more confident prescribing the interventions in session and for homework. They will feel uncomfortable, but check in after the exercise and ask yourself if it was really as catastrophic as you thought it might be.

We have included a medical clearance form at the end of the chapter for you to send to your clients' primary care physicians for approval, which can be helpful if a client has a physical condition you are concerned about prior to starting interoceptive exposures. The exposure exercises listed on the form are the ones most commonly used in panic and agoraphobia treatment. We have also left two blank spots on the form for you to fill in with other exposures you may be using from our ideas throughout this chapter.

## In-Office Exposures: INTEROCEPTIVE EXPOSURES

- **Get hot.** Ask the client to put on several layers including big winter coats, or to sit near a heater or space heater in a small room, to create a sensation of being overheated. This exposure may create other feared sensations as well, such as a feeling of suffocation.

- **Hyperventilate.** Model for the client how to hyperventilate before having your client do this exposure. This involves taking in deep and fast breaths through the mouth and pushing the air back out quickly and forcefully, as if blowing up a large balloon. Have your client do this for one minute.

- **Breathe through a small straw.** Ask your client to breathe through a coffee stirrer or cocktail straw while holding her nose so that there is limited air coming in and out, making it feel as though it is challenging to breathe well. Have the client try to do this exercise for about one minute or longer.

- **Get dizzy.** There are several ways to induce feelings of dizziness. You can ask your client to stand up in the center of the room and start spinning in circles, or she can sit in an office chair that swivels and spin around while in the chair for one minute. You can also ask your client to repeatedly roll her head from side to side for thirty seconds, which can be dizzying.

- **Get up quickly.** Ask your client to sit in a chair and bend forward so her head is near the ground. Have the client stay there for thirty seconds to a minute and then sit up quickly, which can send a rushing feeling to the head.

- **Increase heart rate.** Ask your client to jog in place or repeatedly go up and down a set of stairs for one minute to increase her heart rate.

- **Feel disoriented.** Ask your client to wear someone else's prescription glasses to mimic things looking disoriented and fuzzy.

- **Mimic derealization.** Since clients will report a feeling of derealization when experiencing panic, it is helpful to recreate that sensation as part of interoceptive exposure exercises. We recommend purchasing a strobe light to use in a dark room with your client. You can have the client first practice sitting in the room silently while the strobe light is running, and then later practice having a conversation or doing a routine activity while the light is on so she can learn to continue with routine activities despite feeling anxious. Exposure to flashing lights may be contraindicated in a small percentage of the population, including those who are prone to seizures. You can discuss this with your client prior to beginning the exposure.

- **Have a dry mouth.** Ask your client to put a cotton ball in her mouth to remove saliva and to induce a feeling of dry mouth, which can happen while nervous or panicking.

- **Get tripped out.** Do an online search for "trippy moving circles" or "rotating spirals." Have the client stare at the circles for at least one minute. There are also websites that allow the individual to look at spinning circles followed by pictures of scenes, such as outer space. If the client views the outer space scene (for example) following staring at the moving circles, the outer space scene appears to be moving.

- **Stare at a light.** Ask your client to stare at a fluorescent light in the office for thirty seconds to a minute and then look away and try to read something, such as a magazine or book, which can induce a feeling of derealization.

- **Get caffeinated.** Ask your client to bring a coffee or energy drink with her to session and drink it in a short period of time to feel the effects of the drink.

- **Wear a constricting article of clothing.** Some clients fear getting stomachaches or feeling stomach discomfort. Ask your client to wear a tight belt around the stomach to mimic that uncomfortable sensation. For those who fear the sensation of suffocating or tightness in the throat, you can ask your client to wear a tight scarf around the neck to mimic this sensation.

- **Place a book on the chest.** Ask your client to lie down and place a heavy book on the chest to mimic the sensation of not being able to breathe deeply and freely.

- **Create a nausea jar.** Make a jar with your client of things that smell nasty to her and would create a feeling of nausea, such as cigarette butts, moldy food, or dog poop.

- **Get tense.** Ask your client to hold a push-up position for one minute or as long as possible to mimic the sensation of weak muscles following the feeling of being tense.

- **Tense the throat.** Ask your client to tense her throat in a "mid-swallow" position to induce a feeling of tightness.

## Out-of-Office Exposures: INTEROCEPTIVE EXPOSURES

- **Get caffeinated while in scary places.** Ask your client to drink an energy drink, coffee, or espresso while in a place that is triggering for her panic or agoraphobia, such as while driving or in a crowded store.

- **Hyperventilate.** Ask your client to hyperventilate before entering feared situations, such as a mall or driving, to mimic panic sensations and practice riding out the anxiety out while continuing to engage in everyday activities.

- **Feel uncomfortable in the real world.** Ask your client to practice any of the above interoceptive exposures in real-life scenarios, meaning out of the therapy office. Examples of places to go with the client (or to send her for homework) include the grocery store, the place where she had the first (or scariest) panic attack, work, elevators, or any other feared situations. If you both choose to go to a grocery store, for example, you can sit in the car with the client and have her repeatedly practice these interoceptive exercises and then walk directly into the grocery store. You can also ask her to do some of these within the grocery store.

## Safety Behaviors to Eliminate: INTEROCEPTIVE EXPOSURES

During interoceptive exposures, you want to the client to be fully engaged in the exercise without doing anything to feel safer, such as hyperventilating at a slower pace than you have asked or spinning around slowly. The client may start out strong and then begin to fade the intensity; keep an eye out for this and remind her to pick up the pace. You can even use a metronome or have the client copy your speed in doing the exercise if she has a tendency to "cheat."

When doing interoceptive exposures, we recommend not having the client first know how long she is going to be doing an exercise, as being focused on the clock or counting down the time in her head can become a safety behavior. Use your watch, phone timer, or clock to keep track of the length of the interoceptive exposure exercise without giving the client this information.

Some clients who fear becoming sick will later tell you that they didn't eat or drink prior to coming into the interoceptive exposure session for fear of getting sick. Remind them to keep their dietary routine as normal as possible before coming to therapy, and if there is a snack available and some water, have the client eat or drink before doing the exposure to eliminate the safety behaviors.

## In Vivo Exposures

As discussed in chapter 3, in vivo exposures consist of directly confronting feared situations in real life, as opposed to imagining them. These exposures can be conducted in the office, conducted out of the therapy office with your client, and/or assigned to your client for homework.

Because agoraphobia has a substantial overlap with claustrophobia (in both cases, clients are afraid of becoming trapped and unable to escape), we recommend you review the "Tight Spaces" in vivo exposures in chapter 5. Many can be useful for clients with agoraphobia as well.

### In-Office Exposures: IN VIVO EXPOSURES

- **Say catastrophic thoughts aloud.** Have your client say aloud feared thoughts that are common among those with panic disorder, such as "I am going to suffocate," "I'm losing control," or "I will pass out and be embarrassed."

- **Get locked up.** Lock the client in an area of the therapy office (e.g., closet, court-yard) to target a fear of being "trapped."

- **Limit personal space.** With your client's permission, invite colleagues or trainees into the session and have them stand close to and around the client, or have them also stand in front of the door so that the client does not feel there is an easy way out.

## Out-of-Office Exposures: IN VIVO EXPOSURES

- **Go someplace new.** Give the client directions to a location she has never been to before and have her go there for "homework" without the use of any safety behaviors.

- **Sit in the middle of a row.** Have your client go to a crowded theater, place of worship, or other venue and sit in the middle of the row rather than on the aisle.

- **Wait in line.** Ask the client to wait in line in a store, bank, or coffee shop to target the fear of being in a line. When this becomes easier, ask the client to always choose the longest line at a grocery store or other location.

- **Sit in traffic.** Ask your client to purposefully take a drive during rush hour, regardless of whether she has someplace to go. When the client has multiple route options for how to get to work or another necessary location, ask her to look up the current traffic time for all routes and to choose the busiest one.

- **Take a shopping trip.** Ask your client to go shopping in a mall during peak hours.

- **Take public transportation.** Ask your client to systematically practice riding a bus, subway, or train. Have her start small by going only one stop on the bus or other form of transportation and work up to taking longer trips. Later, you can combine this in vivo exposure with listening to an imaginal exposure script over headphones while on public transportation.

- **Get lost.** Have the client drive you to a location that she is unfamiliar with and that is off the beaten path. Then get out of the car and into either a cab, Uber or Lyft, or the car of a colleague who has been following you, and have the client drive back alone.

## Safety Behaviors to Eliminate: IN VIVO EXPOSURES

Clients with panic disorder and/or agoraphobia may attempt to go to stores or malls during off hours so that they can escape easily if panic-like or embarrassing symptoms arise. This safety behavior should be eliminated as soon as possible. If the client is unable to stop altogether at first, then you can gradually reduce these behaviors. For example, if the client goes to the grocery store only in the early morning because it is less busy, then work toward the goal of getting her to go at 5:00 p.m. after people are getting out of work, or on the weekends. The client may not be ready for this change all at once, so you can arrange for her to try going at lunch time, then at 3:00 one day, then at 4:00, and so on.

## Imaginal Exposures

For feared consequences in which in vivo exposure is not practical, such as when a client with panic and agoraphobia fears throwing up in public, you can use imaginal exposure. As you may remember from chapter 3, imaginal exposure involves creating a story either on paper or on a computer that the client will read aloud (or record on a phone or computer and listen to) repeatedly. You will work with the client to include vivid details that should involve all of the five senses. (See the guidelines in chapter 3 for setting up successful imaginal exposure scripts; we also provide you with an example script at the end of this chapter.)

### In-Office Exposures: IMAGINAL EXPOSURES

- **Write an imaginal exposure script.** Ask your client to write a script about her worst fears related to panic or agoraphobia. (See the example imaginal exposure script at the end of this chapter.) Encourage your client to make a recording of the script so that she can listen to it outside of session or when pairing it with other exposures, such as taking a drive.

- **Read an imaginal exposure script while looking at pictures.** Ask the client to recite or listen to her imaginal exposure script while simultaneously looking at pictures of tight spaces, wide open spaces, or other feared situations.

### Out-of-Office Exposure: IMAGINAL EXPOSURES

- **Read or listen to the imaginal exposure script outside of session.** Many times the imaginal exposure script ends up having the most impact when the client pairs it with doing an in vivo exposure (see earlier lists in this chapter).

### Safety Behaviors to Eliminate: IMAGINAL EXPOSURES

Clients may be inclined to leave out their worst fears and/or very descriptive details while writing the imaginal exposure script. Make sure you are checking in with your client to make sure this is not the case, and if it is, have the client add these details.

# CONCLUSIONS

In this chapter we differentiated between panic attacks and panic disorder and discussed how significant avoidance leads to agoraphobia. We also highlighted the differences between specific phobias and panic/agoraphobia—an important distinction. In vivo, imaginal, and interoceptive exposures are all central components to the treatment of panic disorder. We recommend doing all three of them in your work with your clients. As a concluding message, remember to fight exposophobia and not avoid interoceptive work, one of the most critical interventions in the treatment of panic and agoraphobia.

In the next chapter, we will outline the diagnostic criteria for social anxiety and provide you with helpful and creative behavioral interventions to treat it.

# CHAPTER RESOURCES

**Reminder:** These resources are also available to download and print from http://www. newharbinger.com/43737.

## Medical Clearance Form

Patient Name: _____ Date of Birth: _____

Your patient is currently engaged in cognitive behavioral therapy (CBT) for anxiety. The primary aim of this treatment is to reduce patients' fear of normal physical sensations (e.g., heart racing, hyperventilation, dizziness) and to reduce their avoidance of feared situations and sensations that are often present in anxiety and related disorders. It is possible that some exercises and exposures to feared situations may not be appropriate for all patients. Therefore, since this patient is under your medical care, please provide your professional opinion regarding the appropriateness of each of the following exercises the patient may be asked to try in therapy. For each item, please check "yes" if this patient is medically cleared to engage in this task or "no" if you do not believe this task is appropriate for the patient, given the patient's current medical status. Thank you.

| Task Description | Medically Cleared? | |
|---|---|---|
| | Yes | No |
| 1. Shake head from side to side for 30 seconds | | |
| 2. Climb stairs for 1 minute or until feel heart beating quickly | | |
| 3. Jog in place for 1 minute | | |
| 4. Hold breath for 45 seconds or as long as able to | | |
| 5. Tense body muscles for 1 minute | | |
| 6. Hold a push-up position for 1 minute | | |
| 7. Spin in place for 1 minute | | |
| 8. Voluntarily hyperventilate for 1 minute | | |
| 9. Breathe through a thin straw for 1 minute | | |
| 10. Stare intensely at a spot on the wall for 2 minutes | | |
| 11. (Other) _____ | | |
| 12. (Other) _____ | | |

Your Name (printed):        _____

Signature:            _____

Date: _____

## Example Imaginal Exposure Script—*Panic and Agoraphobia*

*My new boyfriend has been begging me to go to the movie theater with him to see a new movie on opening night. I can't. I just can't. Even thinking about it my hands are sweaty, my stomach is in knots, and I feel dizzy. I know I am supposed to face my fear, so with some encouragement I decide to go. As we get out of the car to walk up to the theater, I can immediately see the long lines that have begun to form to get the tickets. We stand in line with people in front of me, behind me, and all around me. I'm starting to shake and my stomach hurts. The smell of popcorn in the air is making me sick. I feel the nausea rising and I think, What if I get sick in front of all these people? I know how embarrassing it will be but I try to dismiss the thoughts.*

*Eventually, we make it into the theater. I attempt to rush ahead of the crowd in hopes of getting an aisle seat so I won't be trapped in the middle of the crowd. There are none. The room is already packed. We spot two seats in the middle of an aisle down front. How will I get up and run to the bathroom if I am going to be sick? My hands shake, palms now dripping, and I can barely focus on what my boyfriend is saying to me. I feel disoriented and not myself and the nausea begins to climb. As the lights dim and the movie starts, I try to focus but I can't. All of a sudden, I feel acid in my throat, and I know I will soon be sick. I will never make it out. I have to climb over all these people. I jump up and start pushing past people with vomit building in my throat. Just as I climb over the last person, I vomit all over the floor. Everyone is looking at me, some are laughing, and some are seriously grossed out. I am humiliated.*

# CHAPTER 7

# Social Anxiety Disorder

In this chapter, we discuss diagnostic criteria and important considerations regarding social anxiety disorder, followed by exposure ideas related to fear of performance situations such as public speaking, being observed, and using public bathrooms. We also tackle ways to expose clients to more general social anxiety fears such as meeting new people, starting and maintaining conversations, being embarrassed, and having others observe signs that they may be anxious, such as blushing or sweating.

## WHAT IS SOCIAL ANXIETY DISORDER?

Eleven percent of adults and adolescents have a lifetime history of social anxiety disorder (also called social phobia; Kessler et al., 2012). The *DSM-5* (APA, 2013) outlines the following criteria for social anxiety disorder:

A.   A marked fear of social situations in which the person is exposed to possible social scrutiny.

B.   The person fears he or she will act in a way that causes embarrassment or negative judgment by others, or that he or she will show anxiety symptoms that lead to embarrassment or negative social evaluation.

C.   The feared social situations almost always elicit fear.

D.   The feared social situations are either avoided or are endured with intense fear.

E.   The fear is out of proportion to the actual threat or the sociocultural context.

F.   The fear is persistent (e.g., six months or more).

G.   The fear or avoidance causes significant distress or impairment in functioning.

H.   The fear or anxiety is not related to the physiological effects of a medication, substance, or other medical condition.

I.   The fear or anxiety is not explained by another mental health disorder, such as an autism spectrum disorder or panic disorder.

J.   Should another medical condition be present, such as Parkinson's Disease, the fear and anxiety related to social situations must be clearly unrelated to the medical condition or be excessive in nature.

## Fear and Avoidance in Social Anxiety Disorder

The fears in social anxiety disorder can be very specific, such as a fear of engaging in public speaking, or they can be more generalized, in which daily interactions with others are highly anxiety provoking. Individuals with social anxiety often worry that their anxiety will be apparent to others (e.g., that others will see them blush, sweat, or shake) and that they will be judged negatively for appearing anxious. For example, someone with social anxiety may fear going to a cafeteria out of concern that he will drop the tray on the ground, which will cause everyone to look and laugh. Someone else with this fear may worry about stuttering through a presentation in class and everyone in the school laughing or gossiping about what happened. People with social anxiety disorder typically avoid feared situations like these when possible, or endure them with significant distress (and often safety behaviors) if they cannot be avoided. So, for example, the individual who fears dropping his tray at the cafeteria might avoid going to the cafeteria, opting instead to bring lunch from home. The student who is afraid of presentations may spend the class time hiding out in the bathroom or playing "hooky" from school.

## Important Considerations in the Treatment of Social Anxiety Disorder

It is important to note that some individuals with social anxiety have social skill deficits. These deficits can result from going years without having real-life exposure to conversations, attending parties, or speaking in classes, which can lead the individual to fall behind in mastering normative social skills. Therefore, a subset of clients will benefit greatly from social skills training in addition to exposure. Briefly, social skills training involves identifying problems in both verbal and nonverbal aspects of social behavior, and then role-playing social situations using the following steps:

- Giving direct instructions about the social skill (e.g., "I'd like you to try increasing your eye contact.")

- Modeling the appropriate social skill (e.g., taking the client's place in the role-play while demonstrating appropriate eye contact)

- Having the client practice (e.g., doing the role-play while you monitor the client's eye contact)

- Giving direct feedback (e.g., about strengths and weaknesses in eye contact or other verbal or nonverbal aspects of social behavior)

- Repeating as needed

Another important consideration is that social anxiety can create significant interference in everyday life, with negative effects on various activities at school or work, such as communicating with others, giving presentations, participating in discussions or meetings, and forming and maintaining relationships with others. Individuals with social anxiety may try to control their anxiety by self-medicating with alcohol or drugs as a means of avoidance. We recommend you assess this carefully prior to beginning treatment for social anxiety disorder.

# BEHAVIORAL TREATMENT FOR SOCIAL ANXIETY DISORDER

In this chapter, we have divided the in-office and out-of-office exposure ideas for social anxiety disorder into the following categories:

1. Performance-related fears

    a.   Being the center of attention (e.g., giving a speech)

    b.   Using public restrooms

2. Fear related to social situations

3. Fear of embarrassment

    a.   Embarrassing one's self

    b.   Appearing anxious to others

While we provide lists of exposures in this chapter to help your client face his fears related to social situations, performances, using public restrooms, and being embarrassed, it will be important (as always) for you to look for any other factors that contribute to the client's fear in given situations. You can then incorporate these factors into any exposure to make it either more or less challenging, such as talking to individuals of the same sex or different sex, same age or different age, one person or multiple people, and so on. Since the client with social anxiety often fears doing things around others, it can be helpful to gather confederates (such as colleagues or students), when available, to be part of exposures. We recognize that this might not be feasible for many providers in independent practice. Therefore, consider going outside of the office to stores or other places where you can have your client practice interacting with others. We also provide a variety of imaginal exposure scripts for you to use with your client as templates, which you can modify in order to target your client's idiosyncratic fears effectively.

## Performance-Related Fears

There are two main categories of performance-related fears experienced by people with social anxiety disorder: fears of being the center of attention and fears of using public restrooms. The first category consists of a fear of doing something in front of others where the individual is the center of attention, such as giving a presentation or speech, or being on stage. For many (though not all) clients, it is scarier to be observed by a group than by an individual. In such cases, although it will be useful to have the client present or give a speech to you, it will eventually be helpful for him to do those same exposures in front of larger crowds. If you work in a setting where you do not have the option of including others in the exposure, you can ask your client to bring family members or friends to exposures so that he has a larger audience. Consider investing in virtual reality (VR) equipment, as some programs come with "virtual audiences" for giving speeches or being interviewed for a job.

Fears of using public restrooms in social anxiety disorder usually take one of two forms. The first, sometimes called "shy bladder syndrome," reflects a real or perceived inability to urinate around other people who are also using the restroom. Clients with this fear are concerned that others will hear that they aren't urinating and judge them negatively for this. These concerns lead to feelings of anxiety and associated physiological arousal, which can actually tighten the urethral sphincter and make it more difficult to urinate, thus creating a vicious cycle. The second form of public restroom fears reflects concerns that one will make disgusting noises due to urination, flatulence, or defecation and that others will hear these noises.

Below we provide exposures for both types of social anxiety disorder.

# Exposures for Fear of Performing/ Being the Center of Attention

## In-Office Exposures: PERFORMING/BEING THE CENTER OF ATTENTION

- **Use imaginal exposure.** Write a detailed imaginal exposure script of either performing in a show or giving a speech in front of a large group, and it not going well. (See the example script at the end of the chapter.)

- **Use virtual reality.** Use VR equipment so that your client has an "audience" to perform to. With some VR equipment, you can upload an actual speech or presentation that the client needs to give in real life, which can be helpful to target anxiety around an upcoming presentation or talk at work, at school, or in some other area of the client's life.

- **Present on a well-known or easy topic.** Ask your client to begin by giving a one-minute presentation to you alone, and then make the exposure more challenging by increasing the time to five and then ten minutes. The presentation can be on any topic that the two of you choose (e.g., vacations, favorite movies or television shows). You can also ask the client to bring in prepared school or work presentations to use. The client can use slides during the presentation at first, but when that no longer elicits marked fear, you can ask your client to present by memory to make the exposure more challenging.

- **Present on a challenging topic.** Give the client a topic to prepare a presentation on for an upcoming session. Assigning a topic that you know a lot about can be particularly challenging because it also targets the client's fear of presenting when not knowing as much as the "audience." You can give the client feedback following the presentation, and you can also make it harder by having the audience give some harsh feedback (having discussed this in advance with the client). For example, you or other audience members can say, "That really wasn't a good presentation" or "I'm surprised that you didn't seem to put much work into your talk."

- **Have a debate.** Set up a mock debate on a controversial topic, such as the death penalty or abortion. You can bring in confederates (e.g., colleagues or students) to the debate to make the exposure more advanced.

- **Create a mock job interview.** Practice having your client do a job interview with you or a colleague. To make this more realistic, you can ask your client to dress up for the "interview." You can also have the client sit in your waiting room and then go out and bring him back to your office as if it were a true interview. Go through several questions with the client, such as "What are your strengths and weaknesses?" "When was a time there was conflict with a colleague, and how it was resolved?" "Is there anything else you think may be pertinent?" Give feedback at the end of the interview so that he can work to improve certain areas.

- **Brag to others.** Ask your client to prepare a talk called "My Personal Strengths" and to give several examples of times in which he has really excelled. People with social anxiety often do not like to talk about themselves or to bring attention to themselves in any way, which is why this can be a particularly helpful exposure.

- **Put on a show.** Bring your client outside of the office into a waiting room or parking lot and ask him to sing a song (e.g., "Twinkle, Twinkle, Little Star," "Santa Claus Is Coming to Town," or any song of his choosing).

- **Give a speech to an uninterested audience.** Ask your client to give a speech or presentation while you (and confederates, such as colleagues or students, if possible) look bored, play on your phones, and roll your eyes at information that the client provides. The audience of confederates can then ask the client questions, starting with easy ones and then increasing the difficulty level (e.g., "What research can you cite that supports your point on X?").

- **Make mistakes on purpose.** Ask your client to give a speech or presentation while making mistakes on purpose. There can be spelling errors on the slides, or he can plan to mispronounce words or even give incorrect information to the audience on purpose (without telling the audience these mistakes are deliberate, of course).

- **Create an online video.** Encourage your client to post an audition tape, speech, poem, or song online (e.g., Facebook, Instagram, YouTube, SoundCloud) to draw attention to the performance.

## Out-of-Office Exposures: PERFORMING/BEING THE CENTER OF ATTENTION

- **Be on stage.** Visit an auditorium or other setting with a stage. Have the client stand on stage without an audience to get used to the environment. Then have the client start a speech or a monologue with no one in the room but you. If possible, gradually add more people to the room to create a bigger audience.

- **Volunteer to perform.** Ask your client to volunteer to give a presentation, make an announcement at a meeting, or do a reading in a church or other place of worship.

- **Join Toastmasters.** Go online to find a nearby Toastmasters meeting group for your client to join. Toastmasters is a group that allows individuals to practice speaking in front of others to gain confidence in doing so. The client will also get tips for improving his public speaking skills. You can start by having your client sign up and go to a meeting without participating as a beginning step of the process. For some clients, just signing up and attending can be a valuable exposure!

- **Go on a job interview.** Whether or not the client is looking for a job, he can practice interviewing for jobs.

- **Sing karaoke.** Have your client go to a karaoke bar and sing a song on stage with a supportive family member or friend. Later, you can encourage your client to get on stage alone at a karaoke bar. Ask the client to sing a well-known song at first and then later possibly perform something a little more dated or bizarre that an audience might not like as much.

## Safety Behaviors to Eliminate: PERFORMING/BEING THE CENTER OF ATTENTION

Clients may tend to overrehearse their presentations, speeches, or other performances. Help them reduce these behaviors systematically. You can ask them to give "off the cuff" presentations so that there is little time to rehearse. You can also have them set a time for how long they will be allowed to prepare their work for the exposure (or real-life situation).

Individuals with social anxiety often attempt to avoid eye contact with others. Have your client practice making eye contact with you, and then increase the length of the eye contact. Encourage the client to begin practicing increasing eye contact in everyday life as well.

Encourage your client to refrain from looking down or looking at notes excessively during an exposure by setting goals as to how many times he will look up during the exposure.

# Exposures for Fear of Using Public Restrooms

## In-Office Exposures: USING PUBLIC RESTROOMS

- **Use the bathroom with someone standing outside.** You or a confederate (a trainee or colleague) can stand outside of the bathroom door while the client uses the restroom. Progress to having the helper knock on the door and ask questions such as "Is anyone in there?"

- **Practice non-urination with someone standing outside.** Many clients fear that they will be unable to urinate in a public bathroom, and that this failure to urinate will be noticed (by the silence) and judged negatively by others. With a helper outside the bathroom door, have the client practice standing at or sitting on the toilet and not urinating. Advance to having the helper knock on the door and ask questions such as "Why aren't you peeing?"

- **Make flatulence sounds with someone standing outside.** Some clients fear using public bathrooms because of a concern that they will make unflattering noises. Have the client mimic these noises by making flatulence sounds with his mouth. Progress to having the helper knock on the door and ask questions such as "What was that noise?"

- **Make an announcement about going to the bathroom.** Ask your client to announce to people that he or she needs to go to the bathroom and then to go directly next to someone using a urinal or stall even if others farther away are free. Make the exposure more challenging by having the client pour a water bottle filled with water into the toilet and then say, "Boy, did I have to go!"

## Out-of-Office Exposures: USING PUBLIC RESTROOMS

- **Use a public restroom.** Have the client identify public restrooms that have varying levels of traffic (e.g., a public library might have a small number of people, whereas a train station might have many more people). For men, have the client practice using both stalls and urinals.

- **Practice non-urination at urinals.** Because clients fear that others will notice that they aren't urinating, the key is to expose them to the potential embarrassment of non-urination. Try to identify urinals with varying threat levels. Most urinals have partitions between them, which may present less of a perceived threat than those that don't. Some public urinals (e.g., at some older sports venues) have "trough"-style urinals, which may present a significant level of perceived threat. Therefore, you may want to start with urinals that are easier and then gradually make the exposure more difficult.

- **Make flatulence sounds from a stall.** As in the in-office exposure, have the client enter a bathroom stall in a public restroom with others around, sit on the toilet, and make flatulence noises with his mouth. An "excuse me" can draw even more attention to the sound.

## Safety Behaviors to Eliminate: USING PUBLIC RESTROOMS

Waiting for the public restroom to completely or partially empty out is a common safety behavior. Instruct the client to do the opposite—try to maximize the "audience" in the bathroom. Also, some clients with shy bladder will load up on fluids before using the restroom in order to make sure they urinate. Because the aim here is to practice *not* urinating, discourage excessive fluid consumption.

## Fear of Social Situations

Many individuals with generalized social anxiety have significant difficulties in everyday interactions with others. These individuals may avoid making small talk with others, dating, and being in situations where they might bump into people they know, such as stores. Ask the client to pay attention to what happens before and during these social situations and report back to you. For example, perhaps the client went to a party but didn't talk to anyone, or drank alcohol before going on a date. This information will help you tailor future exposures accordingly.

## Exposures for Fear of Social Situations

### In-Office Exposures: SOCIAL SITUATIONS

- **Find a restroom.** Ask your client to go to the waiting room area of your office and ask someone who is walking by or sitting in the office where to find the restroom (even if your client knows where it is and even if it is obvious where it is located).

- **Start a conversation.** Have your client initiate conversation with you in session. If you have others in your office space who can help, it will be useful to have your client practice with them as well.

- **Keep a conversation going.** Have your client practice maintaining conversations. You can reduce your friendliness during an exposure and act withdrawn, giving the client an increasing level of responsibility for keeping the conversation going.

- **Make deliberate blunders.** Ask your client to stutter, drop papers, or tremble on purpose during a conversation with you or with a confederate.

- **Play a small-talk game.** Play a game with your client (and other colleagues, if available) in which the client chooses a topic and a time frame to aim for when talking with others. See rules of the game at the end of this chapter.

## Out-of-Office Exposures: SOCIAL SITUATIONS

- **Connect with new people.** Ask your client to consider going on a date with someone from a dating website or joining a Meetup group in the local area. The first homework assignment might include just signing up for one of these sites. Later, encourage the client to chat with people on the website, eventually working up to going to a group activity or on a brief date (e.g., going for coffee as opposed to going out for dinner).

- **Ask for directions.** Have your client ask a stranger where to find the nearest bathroom or other place. Have him do this several times and record experiences to see how others tended to react when questioned about where to find a location.

- **Attend a party.** Ask your client to go to a small party or gathering to which he was recently invited, and then later go to larger ones (or go alone without friends or family members if that is something that has been challenging in the past).

- **Host a party.** Have your client host his own party or small gathering, if this is something that the client has previously avoided, and invite some people he does not know well and who could potentially turn down the invitation.

## Safety Behaviors to Eliminate: SOCIAL SITUATIONS

Watch out for the following safety behaviors: (1) finding ways to avoid speaking to authority figures such as bosses, teachers, and police officers, (2) avoiding eye contact during conversations or interactions with others, and (3) subtle safety behaviors, including carrying around a phone or other item in order to look busy and thus avoid social encounters. Some adolescents with social anxiety use location maps on Snapchat to see who may be nearby, and then they intentionally avoid those areas. Encourage your client to refrain from these behaviors. Additionally, your clients might speak with others but do so in a quiet voice so that it will not be as apparent if they make a mistake. Therefore, encourage your clients to practice speaking in a louder and more confident voice.

Many socially anxious clients self-medicate by using benzodiazepines, beta-adrenergic blockers, alcohol, or other substances prior to social encounters, or drink alcohol in social situations. Encourage your client to try these exposures without such substances. We recommend you carefully assess substance use in your clients with social anxiety disorder.

## Fear of Embarrassment

Since a fear of embarrassment is a core element of social anxiety disorder, it is essential to target this fear by having your client engage in exposures that lead to (or could lead to) a feeling of being embarrassed. The goal is not to humiliate your clients during an exposure, but rather to have them come in contact with the fear to a degree that would be manageable for someone without social anxiety. We have divided this section into a fear of embarrassing one's self and a fear of appearing anxious to others, either by blushing, sweating, or showing some other sign of outward of anxiety. Note that these exposures can be combined with the other exposures in this chapter—for example, giving a speech (performance-related exposure) while appearing sweaty (embarrassment-related exposure).

## Exposures for Fear of Embarrassment

### In-Office Exposures: EMBARRASSMENT

- **Wear clothes inside out.** Have your client walk around the office with an item of clothing inside out or backward. Consider asking the client to wear two different shoes or socks to draw more attention from others.

- **Ask a silly question.** Have your client ask where the nearest bathroom is while standing in front of the bathroom.

- **Toilet paper trail.** Ask your client to tape some toilet paper to the bottom of his shoe and walk around with it.

- **Double (or triple) check appointment time.** Ask your client to call a doctor's office to confirm the time and date of an upcoming appointment at least twice in a short period of time (e.g., within an hour). At the second call, the client can say something like "I know you told me, but I forgot; can you repeat the date and time of that appointment?"

- **Walk backward.** Ask your client to leave the office and go into the waiting room while walking backward to draw attention.

- **Say hello or goodbye using the wrong name.** Introduce your client to a colleague in your office and then have the client say goodbye using the wrong name. For example, you can introduce the client to "Cindy" and have it prearranged with your client to say, "It was nice meeting you, Mindy" at the end of the conversation.

## Out-of-Office Exposures: EMBARRASSMENT

- **Walk backward.** Have your client walk backward in the mall, in a store, or on a sidewalk to draw unwanted attention.

- **Pay with change.** Either go with your client to a store or ask the client to go alone and pay for an item with only coins (make sure the client doesn't count the coins out ahead of time).

- **Eat alone.** Ask your client to go to a restaurant and eat alone. Start with easier places such as fast food chains and then make it more challenging by asking the client to dine alone in sit-down restaurants.

- **Ask a silly question.** Ask the client to go into a coffee shop and ask the barista if coffee is served there.

- **Drop an item that makes a loud noise.** Have your client drop books on the floor or coins from a pocket or purse, which will make a loud noise and draw attention.

- **Spill a drink.** Ask your client to go to a cafeteria, restaurant, or food court and get a cup of water and then "accidently" spill it on the floor. You can also give your client a cup of water and ask him to go back out to the waiting room and spill the drink on the floor in front of others.

- **Make a return to a store.** Have your client make a purchase in a store and then go back right away and return it.

- **Be wrong.** Encourage your client to answer a question incorrectly in class or in a meeting if it would not be harmful to do so.

- **"Forget" money when checking out.** Encourage your client to get groceries or other items in a store and when checking out, tell the cashier the money is in the car and leave to get it.

- **Have a family member draw attention to the client in public.** Ask a family member of the client to help set up an exposure to embarrass the client in public (with prior permission), such as singing to the client while on an escalator in the mall where many shoppers are present and can see.

- **Wear something goofy.** Encourage your client to visit a public place, such as a shopping mall, while wearing a novelty hat or an attention-getting T-shirt.

## Safety Behaviors to Eliminate: EMBARRASSMENT

Some individuals with social anxiety apologize profusely to others as they do not want to offend anyone. Many times these apologies will be for very minor things that do not require an apology. One goal will be to eliminate excessive apologies to others. Additionally, often clients with social anxiety will make qualifying statements to others about why they are returning things to stores, why they dropped an item, or why they were wrong about something, in order to try to lessen their anxiety. For example, a client might make a return to the store but make an elaborate excuse about why he is returning it rather than just returning it. Ask clients to do these exposures without the qualifying statements.

Watch for avoidance of making eye contact with others and help the client start making eye contact again by practicing with you and then with others.

Clients might be doing the exposures that you asked them to, but during times when stores or other areas are less crowded so that there is a lower chance of being embarrassed or having others see them. Watch out for this and ask your clients if they tend to let anxiety dictate when they do the exposures rather than doing them at a time that maximizes the exposure.

Some fearful clients take medications, such as benzodiazepines or beta-adrenergic blockers, or use alcohol prior to giving a speech or being the center of attention where they might feel embarrassed. Encourage your client to try these exposures without such substances, choosing instead to feel the fear and allow it to come back down on its own.

# Exposures for Fear of Appearing Anxious

## In-Office Exposures: APPEARING ANXIOUS

- **Get sweaty.** Have your client put water on his forehead, under his arms, or on other areas of clothing (e.g., back of shirt, collar) to mimic looking sweaty and then walk around the office space or the parking lot so that others may see that the client is "anxious." Make this exposure more anxiety provoking by pairing it with giving a speech or having a conversation with someone so that the sweaty look is more likely to be noticed.

- **Stutter.** Ask your client to stutter on purpose while speaking with someone else.

- **Look shaky.** Ask your client to appear shaky to others by moving his hands and jiggling his legs so that others could potentially see that he is nervous. Even if this is a symptom that happens naturally for the client, ask him to make it more exaggerated to really come into contact with this fear and make it apparent to others.

- **Wear makeup to look anxious.** Have your client put blush on his cheeks to look flushed and anxious.

- **Use a confederate.** Have a confederate point out to the client how nervous he appears by saying something such as "Wow, you are really sweating! Are you okay?" or "I've never seen you look so shaky before."

## Out-of-Office Exposures: APPEARING ANXIOUS

- **Do the in-office exposures listed above in public places.** Have your client go to work, school, or other public places (e.g., running errands, going to the grocery store) while using the above ideas to target fear of looking anxious (e.g., being shaky on purpose, wearing blush, looking sweaty on purpose).

## Safety Behaviors to Eliminate: APPEARING ANXIOUS

Some clients will have a prescription for a beta-adrenergic blocker so that they will not experience physiological signs of anxiety. Encourage the client to practice doing exposures without having taken the medication beforehand. Additionally, make sure your client isn't using alcohol or drugs to help get through an exposure or make exposures easier.

Ask the client to refrain from apologizing during exposures related to embarrassment, which provides him with temporary relief but is not helpful in the long run. Also, If the client is naturally experiencing blushing, sweating, shaking, or other symptoms, encourage him to continue with what he was doing, such as sitting in a meeting or going to the store, rather than avoiding it or coming up with an excuse to leave early. Finally, clients might have the tendency to try to rush through the exposure; encourage them to slow it down and really stick with it in full, rather than quickly trying to finish it.

# CONCLUSIONS

The fear in social anxiety disorder is twofold. First, clients who are socially anxious fear specific social and performance situations, such as public speaking, being watched, using public restrooms, and initiating or maintaining conversations. In this chapter, we've provided several ideas for in vivo and imaginal exposure that will help your client confront these feared situations. Second, people with social anxiety disorder are often afraid that they will exhibit outward signs of anxiety, or will make blunders, that will prove embarrassing. Here, we recommend that you address these concerns directly by encouraging the client to tolerate embarrassment by deliberately making errors or mimicking signs of anxiety such as sweating, shaking, blushing, or stuttering. These exercises aim to help the client recognize that even embarrassing social encounters need not be catastrophic.

In the next chapter, we will provide detailed exposures for your clients who have been diagnosed with obsessive compulsive disorder (OCD).

# CHAPTER RESOURCES

**Reminder:** These resources are also available to download and print from http://www .newharbinger.com/43737.

### Example Imaginal Exposure Script—*Performance-Related Fears*

*I get up out of my seat and walk to the front of the room to give my presentation to the audience. The room is quite full, and I feel hot and sticky. My heart feels as though it will pound out of my chest and I begin to feel the sweat pooling under my arms. I attempt to pull up my presentation slides on the big screen, but there is a glitch and I can't get it to work. All eyes are on me and I begin feeling more and more nervous. The room is silent and I try to break the silence by saying, "We are having technical difficulties," but no one offers to help me. They just keep staring at me. I scramble trying to fix my slides as soon as possible. Eventually it is fixed and I can begin, though I am already so worked up from my slides not working that I feel close to panic. I stutter over my words as I begin to speak and notice the audience silently judging me. I try to hold the audience's attention, but I see them becoming bored. Some are looking at their phones while others are making quiet comments to each other. I try to focus on my presentation, but all I can think about is what they all are thinking about me. All of a sudden, the audience members start leaving the room. I try to hold it together but I feel a rush of blood go to my face and I know I must be bright red. I want to run out of the room, but my presentation and career will be ruined.*

## Small-Talk Game

**Materials:**

- Small pieces of paper/index cards/sticky notes

- Writing utensils

- Timer on phone or watch

Write down a list of different topic ideas on small pieces of paper. Examples include weather, sports, TV shows/movies, hobbies, and books. Put all ideas in one pile. In another pile, put lengths of time on separate pieces of paper. Examples include thirty seconds, one minute, two minutes, and so on. You can use and cut up the table provided below or create your own.

Ask your client to choose (without peeking) one card from the topic pile as well as one from the time pile. Set the timer for the length of time chosen and begin the exposure with the topic chosen by the client. You can start by having the client engage in small talk with one or two people and then later ask your client to stand up and give a presentation on the topic that was chosen. Add more complicated topics and longer time frames for more challenging exposures!

| 30 seconds | Hobbies |
|------------|---------|
| 1 minute | Current movies and TV shows |
| 2 minutes | Vacations (e.g., favorite spot or place on bucket list) |
| 3 minutes | School/work |
| 5 minutes | Current affairs |
| 7 minutes | Controversial topics (e.g., death penalty, abortion) |

# CHAPTER 8

# Obsessive-Compulsive Disorder

In this chapter, we will give a brief overview of obsessive compulsive disorder (OCD) and provide detailed exposures to help your client who has OCD face her fears of contamination, forbidden or taboo thoughts, fear of causing harm (to self or others), a need for symmetry, and much more.

## WHAT IS OBSESSIVE-COMPULSIVE DISORDER?

OCD is present in approximately 2% of adults (Kessler et al., 2012). According to the *DSM-5* (APA, 2013), the criteria for OCD are:

A. The presence of clinically interfering and distressing *obsessions*, *compulsions*, or both.

*Obsessions* are defined as:

1. Recurrent, persistent, intrusive thoughts that cause marked anxiety or distress.

2. The person attempts to ignore or suppress the thoughts or neutralize them with compulsive behaviors.

*Compulsions* are defined as:

1. Repetitive behaviors or mental acts that the person feels compelled to perform in response to obsessions or according to rigidly applied rules.

2. The behaviors or mental acts are done as an attempt to alleviate the obsessions, to feel less anxious, or to prevent a feared consequence from occurring.

B. The symptoms are time-consuming (e.g., one hour or more per day) or cause significant distress or functional impairment in social, occupational, or other areas of functioning.

C. The symptoms must not be attributable to the physiological effects of a substance, medication, or medical condition.

D.  The disturbance must not be better explained by another mental health disorder (e.g., thought insertion or delusional preoccupations as seen in psychotic disorders).

Obsessions come in many different forms, including worries about touching dirty items, harming oneself or others accidentally or by uncontrollable impulse, having uncomfortable thoughts about religion or sex, or making mistakes.

Compulsions can be visible, such as when someone repeatedly washes her hands or repeatedly seeks reassurance from a loved one. Other times, compulsions can be subtle and not observable to others. Examples of subtle compulsions may include mentally praying, counting, or reassuring oneself that things are okay.

## Fear and Avoidance in Obsessive-Compulsive Disorder

In most cases, individuals with OCD fear some dreaded consequence if they do not perform a compulsive behavior (see Foa, Kozak, et al., 1995). Individuals with contamination-related obsessions often fear contracting a disease if they touch something that seems "dirty." Individuals with harm-based obsessions may fear that they will injure or kill someone, either accidentally (e.g., by hitting them with a car or leaving the oven on) or in response to an uncontrollable impulse (e.g., that they will be seized with the urge to grab a knife and stab someone).

Sometimes, the feared stimulus in OCD is internal to the person. In particular, many clients experience "forbidden" thoughts—for example, the thought I hate God or I want to molest children may intrude into consciousness. In such cases, the person may fear that she will be punished for these thoughts, or that the thoughts signify that she is dangerous, immoral, or crazy.

In some cases, the person with OCD is unable to identify a feared consequence other than prolonged distress. An individual with symmetry-based obsessions, for example, might fear that leaving things uneven will cause a disaster to occur; however, in other cases, the feared consequence may simply be "I will become so upset that I won't be able to stand it and will feel distressed forever."

Avoidance in OCD can be either passive or active. Passive avoidance strategies refer to what the person does not do—for example, the client with contamination fears may refrain from touching anything that appears "dirty." Active avoidance strategies are the compulsions (safety behaviors) in which the person actively tries to "neutralize" fears or obsessive thoughts through an action of some kind—for example, if the client with contamination fears accidentally touches something "dirty," she may feel a need to wash her hands repeatedly. Passive and active avoidance strategies both serve to maintain fear (see chapter 1).

Avoidance can also be either physical or mental. *Physical* avoidance is the avoidance of stimuli external to the person; for example, an individual with harm-related obsessions might avoid being around knives in order to maintain a sense of safety. *Mental* avoidance refers to efforts to avoid thinking obsessive thoughts. For example, when the person with harm-related obsessions has a thought about hurting others, she might try to distract herself, engage in mental rituals, or otherwise attempt to suppress the thought—which often has a paradoxical effect, resulting in thinking about it even more (Tolin, Abramowitz, Przeworski, & Foa, 2002; Wegner, Schneider, Carter, & White, 1987).

## Important Considerations in the Assessment and Treatment of Obsessive-Compulsive Disorder

It's important to assess the client carefully, particularly in cases of harm-related OCD. Some clients are truly suicidal or homicidal, for example, whereas others are plagued with obsessive thoughts about harm to themselves or others. You can make the distinction by examining the extent to which the thoughts are perceived as intrusive or unwanted, and the extent to which they cause emotional distress. Suicidal individuals, for example, deliberately think of harming themselves and often gain a sense of emotional comfort from the thoughts. Individuals with self-harm obsessions, on the other hand, find the thoughts distressing when they arise, and they experience the thoughts as unwanted. Understanding the client's history (e.g., the extent to which they have engaged in harmful behaviors in the past) is another important factor to consider prior to exposure therapy.

Another important consideration in the assessment and treatment of OCD is the onset of a child or adolescent's symptoms. Check in with the parent(s) to see if the child had a sudden and intense onset of symptoms. If so, you should consider the possibility of pediatric autoimmune neuropsychiatric disorder associated with streptococcus, otherwise known as PANDAS (Leonard & Swedo, 2001). This can occur following an infection, such as strep throat. Be aware that other infections can cause similar symptoms, such as Lyme disease, which is attributed to pediatric autoimmune neuropsychiatric syndrome (PANS; Swedo, Leckman, & Rose, 2012). While exposure will still be the treatment of choice for obsessive-compulsive symptoms caused by PANDAS or PANS, it will be important for the child to have bloodwork and/or a throat culture to see if medical interventions are also needed. Therefore, if you suspect these sudden onset symptoms are the result of PANDAS or PANS, refer your client to her primary care provider for further testing and evaluation.

# BEHAVIORAL TREATMENT FOR OBSESSIVE-COMPULSIVE DISORDER

In this chapter, we have divided the in-office and out-of-office exposure ideas for OCD into commonly seen categories of the disorder:

1. Contamination-related fears

2. Scrupulosity-related fears

3. Pedophilia-related fears

4. Harm-based fears (of self and others)

5. Ordering/arranging/"not just right"/symmetry

6. Checking

## Contamination-Related OCD

Contamination-related OCD is one of the most common types of the disorder. This category includes a fear of developing an illness. The fear can be vague, such as thinking, *I will get sick*, or it can involve more specific obsessions of getting an illness, such as *I will contract HIV*. Below is a list of exposures that are aimed to target this fear.

# Exposures for Contamination-Related Fears

## In-Office Exposures: CONTAMINATION

- **The Contamination Macarena.** Whenever you ask clients to touch a contaminated object, you want to make sure they fully engage with the perceived threat by getting the "germs" all over them. OCD, like many other anxiety-related disorders, is famous for "yes-but"-ing the exposures: "Yes, I touched that dirty object, *but* I survived because the germs are only on the tip of my index finger." So, it's important to spread the contamination around. Have your client touch the feared object with his or her entire hand, then rub his or her hands together, and then use both hands to touch his or her clothing, hair, and face, as if dancing the Macarena.

- **Create an imaginal exposure script.** Ask your client to write a detailed exposure script about getting contaminated and becoming extremely ill or dying.

- **Eat foods that others have touched.** Keep a box of crackers, candy, or other small snacks in your office and have the client reach for it and eat from it while reminding her how many people have also eaten from that box and how germy it could be. You can also ask the client to think about what sorts of diseases she may catch from the box of food (e.g., conjunctivitis, stomach bug).

- **Flossing.** Floss your teeth and then hand the floss to your client to touch or hold so that she can come into direct contact with, and "catch," your germs. You can begin by having the client touch part of the floss that wasn't in your mouth (such as the end of the floss) and then later touch all parts of the floss that were "contaminated."

- **Eat fruits or vegetables.** Have your client eat fruits or vegetables without washing them first. Talk to your client about how many people might have touched those foods in the grocery store. Discuss the fact that pesticides may be covering the fruit and that these pesticides are now entering the client's body.

- **Shake hands.** Bring your client around the office and introduce her to people, with the aim of shaking hands with others. This targets the client's fear of becoming contaminated, as well as a fear of accidentally contaminating or harming others. For clients with a fear of contaminating others, "contaminate" the client's hands prior to the exposure by having her touch things that she considers to be dirty or dangerous, such as cleaning supplies.

- **Germ spreading.** Have a "sneezing contest" (without covering the sneeze with your hand) in the office with your client and any others (e.g., colleagues, family members of client). Give awards to the person with the most realistic sneeze and the person who has the sneeze that travels the farthest.

- **More germ spreading.** Have the client touch a "contaminated" object and then prepare food for others without washing her hands, as long as it is reasonably safe to do so.

- **Eat food off of the floor.** Drop a snack onto the floor for your client and then have her eat it. Begin by using food items that may not collect as many germs or dirt on them, such as a cracker, but then later drop more challenging items such as a piece of cheese or some peanut butter, which is more likely to have stuff on it after being on the ground. Have the client brush off any visible dirt, then eat the snack.

- **Touch doorknobs.** Walk around the office space with your client and have her touch all doorknobs in the building (make sure the palm of the hand comes into contact with the door). This exposure, like all touching-related contamination exposures, can be intensified using "The Contamination Macarena" described above.

- **Sit on the bathroom floor.** Sit on the bathroom floor with your client and go back and forth talking about all the types of germs that may now be on your pants and other parts of your body.

- **Sit on a public bathroom seat.** Ask your client to use the bathroom in your office or another public space without putting down toilet paper first.

- **Touch items in a public bathroom.** Have your client flush the toilet with her hands, as opposed to using a foot or toilet paper. You can then instruct your client to touch the toilet seat and then touch her clothes, or face, or hair.

- **Trash touching.** Have the client touch outside parts of a trash can without gloves or other protective material. To later make the exposure more challenging, you can have the client reach into a trash can and touch items inside or rub her hands on the trash can lining.

- **Touch bodily fluids.** Have the client use toilet paper to collect a microscopic sample of urine, feces, semen, or other "dirty" bodily fluids, then practice touching the paper and spreading the contamination.

- **Eat in the bathroom.** Eat while sitting on the bathroom floor, using the toilet seat as a table.

- **Play games with contaminants.** Especially (though not exclusively) for young people with OCD, it can be useful to adapt games to incorporate contaminants. For example, you could play a game of catch using a raw meatball, play checkers using dead cockroaches, or have a squirt gun fight in which the water has been "contaminated" with a drop of urine or blood.

## Out-of-Office Exposures: CONTAMINATION

- **Get dirty.** Encourage the client to cover her hands with dirt from outside and to get the dirt in between the fingers and under the fingernails.

- **Go on a scavenger hunt.** Have your client go on a hunt to pick up trash in the neighborhood or office complex to do a good deed! Tell you client to consider having a snack afterward (without washing her hands).

- **Dumpsters.** Have the client go outside your office building or to other buildings to touch dumpsters (hospital dumpsters may be rated as even higher-level exposures by clients). She can start by standing near the dumpster, touching the outside of the dumpster, touching the inside of the lid, and then putting her hand inside of the dumpster.

- **Use public transportation.** Ask the client to hold onto the pole in a subway without wearing gloves or other protective gear.

- **Be with others who could be sick.** Have your client sit in a waiting room at a physician's office or hospital, where many sick individuals will be walking in and out. Depending on how busy the waiting room is, you can have the client think about or talk with you about the various illnesses that could be floating around the hospital or doctor's office that have now "contaminated" the client.

- **Bottle up contaminants.** Ask the client to put "contaminants" into a spray bottle and carry the bottle around with her, spreading the contaminants. For example, the client could have a family member cough or sneeze into the bottle first and then spray "clean" things (e.g., interior of car, keyboard of laptop, cell phone) to contaminate them.

- **Make or buy a contamination object.** Have the client make (using online tutorials) or buy slime, putty, or playdough and then contaminate it by bringing it into the bathroom and touching the floor or toilet with it. The client should carry the slime, putty, or playdough around and/or play with it throughout the day and week.

- **Wear a contamination necklace.** Ask your client to contaminate an item that she can wear on a necklace or lanyard around the neck; this way the contaminated object will be close to the face and therefore may be perceived as more likely to get her sick. The client can contaminate items by bringing them into the bathroom, rubbing them on the floor, having others touch them, or putting them in the dirt.

- **Be in close proximity to chemicals.** Encourage your client to keep an open bottle of a "toxic" chemical around, such as on the bedside table or near food.

- **Eliminate "clean" zones.** Many individuals with contamination-related OCD have "clean" and "dirty" zones in their homes. The "clean" zones are areas from which the client has prevented the entry of contaminants. Encourage the client to wear contaminated clothes or bring other items that are considered "dirty" into the clean zones of the home, thus eliminating the "clean" zones altogether.

## Safety Behaviors to Eliminate: CONTAMINATION-RELATED FEARS

Many clients will wear protective gear such as gloves or use the sleeve of a shirt when touching "contaminated" objects, but this will greatly interfere with the learning process, so encourage them to remove these protective barriers. Also, check in with the client to make sure that she does not have friends or family members participating in compulsions (e.g., opening doors so that the client does not have to touch them).

Clients will have an urge to wash or use hand sanitizer after touching "contaminated" objects. However, this behavior will serve to "undo" the exposure, especially if the client is only getting through the exposure by knowing that she can wash later. Gently remind the client that we wouldn't want to undo all of the hard work she just did in session or for homework. This can help motivate her to stick with the uncomfortable feelings without engaging in compulsive behavior. Check in with your client to make sure that she client does not take excessively long showers, or shower frequently throughout the day, as a way to alleviate anxiety; help the client reduce the amount of time in the shower each day until the client is completely abstaining from this safety behavior, meaning that she might not be showering for days.

Some clients may touch or sit in public spaces but then make sure that they don't touch certain areas of their home or car in an effort to prevent contamination and to keep certain places "clean." Clients with contamination-related OCD often have "clean zones" and "dirty zones." They often keep the "clean zones" pristine from outside contamination. For example, some clients will have certain clothes that they believe are okay to be worn in the house as they are deemed "clean," while other clothes are allowed to be worn out of the house but then cannot be worn in the home for fear of contaminating the "clean" rooms of the home. Make sure to check in with your client about this and remove these behaviors as soon as possible as they only serve to maintain the anxiety in the long term. Encourage the client to spread contamination to the "clean zones." Remember, "clean" is the enemy!

## Scrupulosity-Related OCD

Another common type of OCD includes scrupulosity-related fears of not being moral enough, offending a religious figure or religion, or having preoccupations about sex, sexuality, or violence. We begin this section of exposures by tackling the fear of offending a religious figure or of not acting morally enough. This can be a tricky type of OCD, as you need to be sensitive to the client's religious beliefs. It is helpful to have a conversation with your client about her religious beliefs *without* OCD being part of the picture. This will help you discern what is a religious belief and what is an OCD thought or behavior, which you can then challenge. The goal is never to get a client to change her religious beliefs. If needed, you can ask for permission to contact the client's minister, rabbi, or priest for additional guidance or assistance.

# Exposures for Scrupulosity-Related Fears

## In-Office Exposures: SCRUPULOSITY-RELATED FEARS (RELIGION)

- **Draw pictures.** Have your client draw a picture of the devil (or other feared being) or print a picture of the devil from the Internet and color it in, while repeatedly stating the feared outcome, such as "I could go to hell for drawing this."

- **Imaginal exposure.** Create an imaginal exposure script to target the client's worst fear, such as doing something to upset God or a religious figure and the consequences of it (e.g., dying, going to hell, or being punished in other ways).

- **Make a spirit board (popularly known as a Ouija board).** With the client, create a spirit board out of cardboard and printed letters to be glued onto the board (see "Chapter Resources" at the end of this chapter for a description, instructions, and a template).

- **Say feared statements aloud.** Depending on the client's fears, have the client make statements repeatedly such as "I hate God," "I am sinful," or "I will burn in hell."

- **Use Pig Latin.** Have the client say prayers or other ritualistic phrases in "Pig Latin" in order to break up the ritual and potentially offend the higher power. For example, if the client repeatedly says, "God, please keep me safe," this would be translated to "Odgay, easeplay eepkay emay afesay."

- **Rip up a book.** Get a religious book or hymnal and have the client tear pages out of it.

- **Read the Bible in the bathroom.** Bring the Bible or other religious text into a bathroom so that it becomes "contaminated" and could offend God or a religious figure.

- **Fake tattoos.** Draw "666" in black marker on the client's arm and have her wear it around all day. To make it even more challenging, have the client enter a place of worship with that on underneath her clothes.

- **Pray to the devil.** With the client, light a candle and ask for the devil to take your souls. You can use this popular Satanic prayer:

> *Our Father, who art in hell*
> *Cursed be thy name*
> *Thy kingdom upon earth has come*
> *Thy will be done in hell as it is on earth*
> *Grant us your power and might*
> *And lead us into temptation*
> *Deliver us unto evil*
> *Thine is the kingdom of earth*
> *The power and the glory*
> *Forever and ever*
> *So it is done.*

## Out-of-Office Exposures: SCRUPULOSITY-RELATED FEARS (RELIGION)

- **Carry "bad" pictures.** Have your client secretly carry pictures of the devil, a well-known murderer, or other "bad" beings or people into a religious building.

- **Think "bad" thoughts.** Have the client think "bad" thoughts (e.g., curse words, sexual content) while in a church or other religious building.

- **Buy a devil figurine.** Ask your client to place an order online for a devil figurine and then leave it in her bedroom or on her desk at work. You can later make this exposure more challenging by having the client pray to the devil figurine and say aloud that she follows this devil figurine.

- **Try to contact spirits.** Ask the client to purchase a Ouija board or bring a spirit board that she made in session into her home.

- **Take communion "incorrectly."** Have the client drop a piece of the communion wafer or take it a little bit earlier or later than is normally done in the specific place of worship where the client attends.

- **Have nonkosher food nearby.** If the client is keeping kosher, you can ask her to have nonkosher food in the vicinity of the other food that she will eat, without actually eating the nonkosher food.

## Safety Behaviors to Eliminate: SCRUPULOSITY-RELATED FEARS

Make sure that the client isn't praying excessively or saying any prayers that serve to "undo" exposures. Also, some clients will want to seek reassurance from God or another religious figure following an exposure; encourage the client to resist this urge. Finally, work to eliminate any safety behaviors that consist of excessively confessing, either to friends or family or to a priest, rabbi, or minister.

## Pedophilia-Themed OCD

Some clients with OCD have frightening thoughts that they are (or will become) a pedophile or will engage in sexual acts with children. How is this different from pedophilia, and how can you tell the difference between the two? There are several features that differentiate the two disorders, as shown in table 3.

### TABLE 3. Differences between pedophilia-themed OCD and pedophilia

|  | Pedophilia-Themed OCD | Pedophilia |
|---|---|---|
| *Frequency and intensity of thoughts* | Very frequent, intrusive, and distressing | Less frequent, voluntary, and gratifying |
| *Content of thoughts* | Fear of sexual attraction to children | Sexual attraction to children |
| *Behavioral response to thoughts* | No action on thoughts<br><br>Avoids triggers, minimizes contact with children | Action on, or masturbation toward, thoughts<br><br>Seeks out children or child-related stimuli, engages in grooming behavior |
| *Cognitive response to thoughts* | Thought suppression | Fantasizing |
| *Presence of other OCD symptoms* | Common | Less common |

As shown in the table 3, individuals with pedophilia-themed OCD experience sexual thoughts about children as being frequent, intrusive, and distressing. They are characterized by a *fear* of being sexually attracted to children, rather than an actual sexual attraction toward children (see Bruce, Ching, & Williams, 2018; Veale, Freeston, Krebs, Heyman, & Salkovskis, 2009; Vella-Zarb, Cohen, McCabe, & Rowa, 2017). The anxiety will rise every time they experience a thought such as *What if I looked at that child inappropriately?* or *Did I just feel aroused when seeing that picture of my child's friend?* The individual with OCD begins to question herself and has fears that she is a monster and a terrible person. These intrusive thoughts torment the individual, who may then engage in compulsive behaviors or avoidance behaviors. She may avoid or attempt to avoid children (maybe even her own), or engage in neutralizing behaviors. For example, an individual with these intrusive thoughts may take the long way home from work to avoid driving by a playground filled with children. Or a father may no longer change his child's diaper and instead ask his spouse to do it. This is in stark contrast to pedophilic disorder, described in the *DSM-5* as recurrent, intense sexual fantasies, urges, or behaviors involving sexual activity with a prepubescent child for a period of at least six months and acting upon these urges (APA, 2013). Individuals with this disorder are attracted to young children and will seek out opportunities to prey on children or come into contact with them, such as going to playgrounds, looking at child pornography, or molesting a child. Once we have determined that our client has OCD and not pedophilia, we do not fear using exposure strategies.

## Exposures for Pedophilia-Themed Fears

### In-Office Exposures: FEARS OF BEING/BECOMING A PEDOPHILE

- **Repeating scary phrases.** Ask your client to repeatedly state, "I am a pedophile" or "I am attracted to children."

- **Read stories of sexual abuse by clergy.** Read stories of clergy who engaged in molestation of young children with or to your client. To make the exposure more challenging, you can ask your client to say, "If religious figures could do this, then I am capable of it too."

- **Watch video clips of pedophiles.** Conduct an online search for people who have been arrested for pedophilia who talk about their stories. While watching these clips, have your client repeatedly state, "This could be me" or "I am just like this person."

- **Agree with pedophiles.** Watch clips of known pedophiles who talk about how sinister or sneaky they were to approach children or get them to comply and have your client say, "That was a good idea."

- **Look at swimsuit advertisements.** Conduct an online search with your client for children's swimsuit ads and have your client look closely at the pictures without averting her gaze.

- **Rate attractiveness.** Look up online photos of children and ask your client to rate the sexual attractiveness of the children.

- **Write an imaginal exposure script.** Work with your client to create a detailed imaginal exposure script related to her fears of being attracted to a child, engaging in inappropriate acts, and ultimately being arrested for child molestation.

## Out-of-Office Exposures: FEARS OF BEING/BECOMING A PEDOPHILE

- **Go to previously avoided places.** Ask your client to visit places once avoided, such as to go to a playground with her children again or to drive past schools.

- **Read an imaginal exposure script.** Ask your client to bring her imaginal exposure script to a place where there are children and read it silently or listen to it through headphones while looking at children.

- **Watch a documentary.** Ask your client to watch documentaries with the theme of pedophilia, such as *Leaving Neverland, The Paedophile Next Door,* or *Abducted in Plain Sight.* Your client can make the exposure more challenging by stating feared phrases (e.g., "I am a pedophile," "I am attracted to children") while watching the show.

## Safety Behaviors to Eliminate: PEDOPHILIA-THEMED FEARS

Make sure that the client isn't saying things that serve to "undo" the exposure, such as going through all the reasons why she is not a pedophile. In addition, some clients will want to seek reassurance from others or from the Internet that they are not a pedophile. Your client may be conducting online searches for the differences between OCD and pedophilia on a frequent basis. Work with your client to reduce these reassurance-seeking behaviors.

Work to eliminate any safety behaviors that consist of your client's avoiding normal, everyday activities such as changing her child's diaper, helping the child in the bathroom, or helping the child get dressed for school, which the spouse might have taken over to help alleviate the client's anxiety.

## Harm-Based OCD

Harm-based OCD thoughts can be a fear of harming oneself or others (e.g., significant other, children, random person). The client, of course, does not have a desire to harm herself or others and is highly concerned that it could happen because she is not careful enough. She may also fear that she could randomly act impulsively to harm someone even with no history of this in the past. Naturally, it is crucial that you have diagnosed your client carefully and that it is clear that the client has OCD rather than actual suicidal or homicidal ideation. Table 4 shows some key differences between harm-related OCD and actual suicidal or homicidal ideation. As we saw in the example of pedophilia-themed OCD above, the critical distinction is that individuals with OCD *fear* harming themselves or others, whereas people with suicidal or homicidal ideation *desire* or *fantasize about* harming themselves or others. Of course, it's worth noting that people with OCD can frequently have true suicidal ideation; therefore, careful assessment is critical. We wouldn't want to do suicide-related exposures with a truly suicidal individual; on the other hand, we don't want to treat harm-related OCD thoughts without exposure.

### TABLE 4. Differences between harm-related OCD and suicidal or homicidal ideation

|  | **Harm-Related OCD** | **Suicidal or Homicidal Ideation** |
|---|---|---|
| *Frequency and intensity of thoughts* | Very frequent, intrusive, and distressing | Less frequent, voluntary, dependent on negative emotion, can be comforting |
| *Content of thoughts* | Fear of harming self or others | Desire to harm self or others |
| *Behavioral response to thoughts* | No action on thoughts<br><br>Avoids triggers, such as sharp objects | Planning harm to self or others, or actual harming behaviors |
| *Cognitive response to thoughts* | Thought suppression | Wishing or fantasizing |
| *Presence of other OCD symptoms* | Common | Less common |

# Exposures for Harm-Based Fears—Self

## In-Office Exposures: FEAR OF HARMING SELF

- **Be around knives.** Sit in the office with your client with a knife block on the table. Ask your client to stare at the knives and repeatedly say, "I could grab those knives and stab myself."

- **Watch video clips.** Watch video clips with your client of television shows or movies online that portray people engaging in self-harm and/or talking about it, such as the movies *Girl, Interrupted* and *Thirteen*.

- **Use imaginal exposure.** Write a detailed and gory story with your client about harming oneself and the consequences of that behavior, such as a trip to the emergency room, being locked up in a psychiatric ward, or even death (see the sample imaginal exposure script at the end of the chapter).

- **Hold knives.** Have your client hold a knife block and then start holding different knives within the knife block, starting with a butter knife and working up to a butcher knife. Later you can ask your client to hold a knife while stating, "I'm going to stab/ cut/kill myself." The client can (carefully) hold the knife to her wrist to intensify the exposure.

- **Be around a bottle of pills.** Have your client look at or hold a bottle of pills. Ask the client to repeatedly say, "I'm going to take these and overdose."

- **Confront heights.** With your client, stand by an open window on a high floor or find some other high place to go (see chapter 5 for some examples). Have the client look down and repeat, "I'm going to jump."

## Out-of-Office Exposures: FEAR OF HARMING SELF

- **Watch videos while home alone.** Have your client watch movie clips of individuals who harmed themselves.

- **Be around sharp objects.** Tell the client to have a pair of scissors or a razor lying on the table next to her.

- **Go to a kitchen store.** Have your client visit the knife aisle of a kitchen store or other large store that may have various knives (e.g., butcher knife, bread knife) to see and/or touch. The client may need to begin the exposure with someone else accompanying her and then later should spend time in the aisle alone.

- **Cook with knives.** Ask your client to prepare a meal using various sizes of knives. At first, the client may need to do this while others are home, but then she can advance to cooking with knives while home alone.

# Exposures for Harm-Based Fears—Others

## In-Office Exposures: FEAR OF HARMING OTHERS

- **Use imaginal exposure.** Write a detailed story with your client about harming someone while either driving or being around sharp objects. Make sure to encourage her to add all the gory details as well as the consequences of the harming behavior, such as going to jail. (See the sample imaginal exposure script at the end of this chapter.)

- **Be around knives or other sharp objects.** Sit with your client in the office with a knife block or scissors on the table. Then ask colleagues or friends and family members to join the session so that the client can be around sharp objects and people at the same time.

- **Hold sharp objects.** Have your client hold knives from a knife block or other items, such as scissors. You can later ask your colleagues or friends and family members of the client to be present in the session without having the client touch the others at this point. The client can also say, "I am going to hurt one of you" while holding the sharp object but not make any motion, at this point, toward the others in the room.

- **Say threatening words.** Have the client point any knife (depending on how high up on the hierarchy) at you and repeatedly state, "I'm going to hurt/kill/cut you."

- **Hold sharp objects to others.** Have the client hold a butter knife to your wrist. Increase the intensity of the exposure by later having the client hold more challenging knives such as steak knives or butcher knives to your wrist. You can then create a more challenging exposure in which you ask your client to hold a butter knife (and then later sharper knives, such as a butcher knife) to your neck, maybe starting with touching the side of the neck with the knife and then moving to the front of the neck.

- **Kill people with thoughts.** Stand at the window of your office with your client and have your client try to "kill" people with thoughts. This may be even more challenging with children or elderly people. You can have the client think, *I hope you die* or *I want you to die* as the person walks by. Have the client try to appear mean and menacing, rather than looking scared or anxious, while thinking these thoughts. You can also have the client practice saying this about loved ones such as by saying, "I want _____ to die in a car accident."

- **"Poison" someone.** Have your client stand near chemicals, such as cleaning supplies, in your office and then go into the hallway and have the client offer candy to someone directly from her hand. This will help target the fear that the client could have somehow put chemicals into the candy and contaminated another person.

## Out-of-Office Exposures: FEAR OF HARMING OTHERS

- **Cook with knives.** Ask your client to prepare meals at home using large knives while other people are around.

- **Carry knives around.** Have your client carry knives in public. If needed, the client can start with plastic knives and work up to a sharp pocketknife.

- **Sleep with knives in the bedroom.** Ask the client to sleep with a large knife in the nightstand or near the bed to target the concern that she may grab it impulsively in the night and harm someone.

- **Take a drive.** Have your client drive while someone in the car says, "You are going to hit someone."

- **Run over an object.** Ask the client to drive over a life-size dummy (you can make one out of a long-sleeved shirt and pants, stuffed with foam rubber or similar material) to practice hitting someone. Note that you should do this exposure in a more secluded area to avoid having passersby think someone is actually being run over.

- **Use baby dolls.** Have your client drive slowly around a parking lot while you toss baby dolls at the car so that the client hears the thump of the "baby" hitting the car and sees the "baby" flying off the hood or back of the car. You can also have the client put a doll on the ground and run over it repeatedly with the car.

- **Drive during peak hours.** Have your client drive during rush hour or in busy parking lots. You can also ask others to join the session and stand in various places in the parking lot and slap the car as the client drives by.

- **Carry potentially harmful items.** Have your client carry silicone packets (that often come in shoe boxes or with other items you have purchased) and go to a buffet or salad bar to potentially come into contact with someone else's food while carrying "poison."

## Safety Behaviors to Eliminate: HARM-BASED FEARS (SELF AND OTHERS)

Some clients will have removed all of the knives or sharp objects from the home, so make sure the client is bringing those everyday items back into the home. If the client is having others chop vegetables or use utensils or other sharp items for her, work on having the client do these things again.

To make sure that they did not accidently hit someone with their car, some clients will seek reassurance from friends or family, check the rearview mirror of the car repeatedly to make sure no one is lying on the road, turn the car around to make sure no one was hurt, or check the news to ensure there were no hit-and-run accidents that day that they might have been involved in. Encourage the client to stop these behaviors. Some clients who fear hit-and-run accidents will not drive with music on so that they can hear more clearly if they hit someone. Therefore, ask the client to start playing soft music while driving and work up to having loud music playing while driving. Also encourage clients to refrain from having friends or family members drive them as a way to avoid facing the fear of driving.

## Ordering/Arranging/"Not Just Right"/Symmetry OCD

Some clients with OCD have a concern about having things around them be "just right," doing things a certain way, or repeating actions until their bodies feel a certain way. This has been termed the "not just right experience," or NJRE (e.g., Coles, Frost, Heimberg, & Rhéaume, 2003). The individual with this type of OCD may engage in compulsions that include making sure things are orderly, such as lining up all shoes in the closet the right way, making sure that canned goods are properly lined up and organized, or ensuring that all objects on a desk are placed "just right." Exposures should be designed to disrupt this "just right" experience.

# Exposures for Ordering/Arranging/ "Not Just Right"/Symmetry

## In-Office Exposures: ORDERING/ARRANGING/"NOT JUST RIGHT"/SYMMETRY

- **Use imaginal exposure.** Write a detailed story with your client about things being a mess at home, record it, and have your client listen to it while imagining the mess.

- **Write in a sloppy manner.** Have your client write words on paper or a white board in the office without erasing them or rewriting them to look perfect.

- **Get a fake tattoo.** Draw a fake tattoo on your client's arm or hand (with her permission, or course) of numbers, letters, words, or shapes that are asymmetrical, messy, or misspelled.

- **Take an asymmetrical walk.** Have your client walk around outside your office building with one foot on the sidewalk and one foot on the street.

- **Look at pictures.** Have your client look at pictures online of messy houses or of houses of people with hoarding disorder.

- **Color pictures.** Give your client something to color, such as a coloring book, and have her do it in a messy way that includes going outside of the lines.

- **Mess up your office.** Encourage the client to make a "mess" in your office, such as putting the books on your bookshelf out of order or upside down, tilting your pictures or diplomas on the walls, and so on.

- **Change shoelaces.** Have your client take out one shoelace and lace it back in the shoe incorrectly, such as by skipping holes in the shoe and having the remainder of the shoelace be of different lengths.

## Out-of-Office Exposures: ORDERING/ARRANGING/"NOT JUST RIGHT"/ SYMMETRY

- **Rearrange closet or cabinets at home.** Have the client rearrange closets at home so that clothes or shoes are not lined up properly.

- **Cut food.** Encourage the client to prepare food at home, chopping the food at different lengths and widths. For example, instead of cutting a sandwich in half, have the client cut it so one side has three-quarters of the sandwich and the other has one-quarter of the sandwich.

- **Make a mess in the home.** Have the client deliberately cause chaos in a room of the home.

- **Have someone else make a mess in the home.** Have the client choose a friend or family member to make a mess in a room of the home. Encourage the client to watch the mess being created without changing it.

- **Get dressed in a sloppy way.** Have the client put on clothes and wear them in an uneven way, such as wearing two different socks or shoes, buttoning a shirt incorrectly, or wearing a hairstyle with hair pieces falling out of sections of a braid or ponytail.

- **Hang pictures.** Have the client hang a picture in a crooked position in the bedroom.

- **Change the light bulb.** Have the client take one light bulb out of one of the two bedside table lamps so the lighting is asymmetrical.

## Safety Behaviors to Eliminate: ORDERING/ARRANGING/"NOT JUST RIGHT"/ SYMMETRY

Some clients will fix items around the house to make sure everything is properly aligned. Encourage the client to take pictures of the rooms and the house and show them to you periodically to make sure those behaviors have stopped at home. Also, some clients might avoid rooms or places that are not neat or orderly, such as a messy basement or garage in the home. Have the client purposefully spend time in the rooms or places she has been avoiding.

Additionally, some clients with concerns about orderliness will ask others, such as those who live in the home with the client, to tidy up "just so." Encourage the client to eliminate this behavior. If clients have a cleaning service, encourage them to eliminate or reduce the frequency of visits.

## Checking-Based OCD

The individual who has OCD related to checking behaviors may have concerns about safety that lead her to repeatedly check that the stove is turned off, the water is turned off, or the doors or windows are shut and locked in the house to ensure an intruder won't break into the home. A subset of checking-based OCD involves individuals who have to check and/or re-do what they read or write in order to be certain that it's correct or "perfect."

## Exposures for Checking-Based Fears

### In-Office Exposures: CHECKING

- **Use imaginal exposure.** Write a detailed script with the client about leaving the stove or sink on in her home and the consequences of this error. (See the sample imaginal exposure script at the end of this chapter.)

- **Create uncertainty.** Go into the bathroom or kitchen area of your office with your client and have her turn the water faucet on and off and walk away without knowing whether it was completely turned off or not.

- **Repeat feared phrases about uncertainty itself.** Ask your client to repeatedly state, "I will never know" about her obsessional fear.

- **State the feared outcome aloud.** Should a client be worried about having left the stove on at home, for example, have her repeatedly state, "I left the stove on at home" or "My house could be burned down by now."

### Out-of-Office Exposures: CHECKING

- **Briefly leave the home while the stove is on.** Encourage the client to leave the stove on and go to the mailbox to check the mail. Then have the client increase the amount of time spent out of the home, such as running a brief errand while baking cupcakes.

- **Run errands with the sink on.** Have the client leave the sink dripping and go run an errand close to home; slowly increase the time spent away from the house.

- **Leave appliances on at work.** Ask your client to leave the coffee machine on or faucet running at her place of work.

- **Create uncertainty.** Have your client turn a water faucet, oven, or appliance on and off quickly, and leave the home without checking.

## In-Office Exposures: REREADING AND REWRITING

- **Tackle reading or writing.** Provide a paragraph or story for the client to read in session while refraining from rereading. Alternatively, ask the client to write a brief passage using a pen, rather than a pencil, so that she will be unable to erase mistakes easily. Whether reading or writing, encourage the client to deliberately make "mistakes" such as skipping, misspelling, or mispronouncing words.

- **Make things messy.** Ask the client to write down letters, phrases, and sentences without erasing and rewriting it to make it look "just right." Ask her to then start making it very sloppy on purpose. You can also ask her to write down phrases as messily as she can and then you have to try to read it. You can say, "That handwriting is so messy; I can barely read it" or "You weren't even trying at all here," to help increase the anxiety during the exposure.

- **Give a "quiz."** Choose a paragraph from any book or article and ask the client to read it quickly. You can even set a timer if the client has trouble finishing reading in a given amount of time. You can then "quiz" the client on the material. The client may have an urge to check back again and again in the same paragraph to make sure that she comprehended all of the material and didn't miss anything; discourage this repeated checking.

## Out-of-Office Exposures: REREADING AND REWRITING

- **Make mistakes on purpose.** Have the client do assignments from school or work while making mistakes on purpose. You can print out worksheets from the Internet (e.g., math worksheets) to help the client practice filling things in incorrectly without rewriting.

- **Read while having distractions.** Ask the client to do reading assignments from school or work while experiencing significant distraction, such as while playing loud music through headphones or having the television turned on loudly while continuing to read without rereading.

## Safety Behaviors to Eliminate: CHECKING; REREADING AND REWRITING

For those who repeatedly check things for safety reasons, make sure that the client refrains from having someone else check the stove, locks, or doors (whether or not the client is checking herself).

Some clients whose checking-based OCD pertains to rereading or rewriting will be using a tablet or computer to write things down to make it easier to edit and will avoid pen and paper. Therefore, encourage the use of pen and paper when taking notes or completing homework assignments.

# CONCLUSIONS

Treatment of OCD, as with other anxiety-related disorders, is based largely on the process of exposure. Safety behaviors, which in the case of OCD are known as compulsions, should be eliminated as soon as possible in the process. Exposures to feared contaminants, risky situations, or imperfection are powerful tools in the OCD therapist's repertoire, as are imaginal exposure to "forbidden" religious or sexual thoughts, or to fears of harming one's self or others. In the next chapter, we will provide various exposure ideas for the treatment of different types of traumatic experiences.

# CHAPTER RESOURCES

**Reminder:** These resources are also available to download and print from http://www.newharbinger.com/43737.

## Directions for Making an Elaborate Spirit Board

Items that you will need:

- A piece of cardboard or poster paper

- Glue

- Letters of the alphabet printed out

- Numbers 0–9 printed out

- The words "yes," "no," "hello," and "goodbye" printed out

- Scissors

- A "planchette" (i.e., a small object that is needed for the spirit to write back to you using letters on the board)

A spirit board is a "game" that some say can allow you to come into contact with spirits (either good or bad). In this exposure you will create a board as an attempt to contact a spirit. Sit down together and create a spirit board by gluing cutout letters and numbers onto the board or poster paper. Once it is complete, put your planchette on the board. Place your fingers on the planchette and see if you can communicate with a spirit by asking questions aloud to spirits and seeing if the planchette moves to various letters and numbers to answer your questions.

## Simple Spirit Board

**Directions:** Use the printout provided to try to contact a spirit.

**Item that you will need for the simple board:** A "planchette" (i.e., a small object that is needed for the spirit to write back to you using letters on the board)

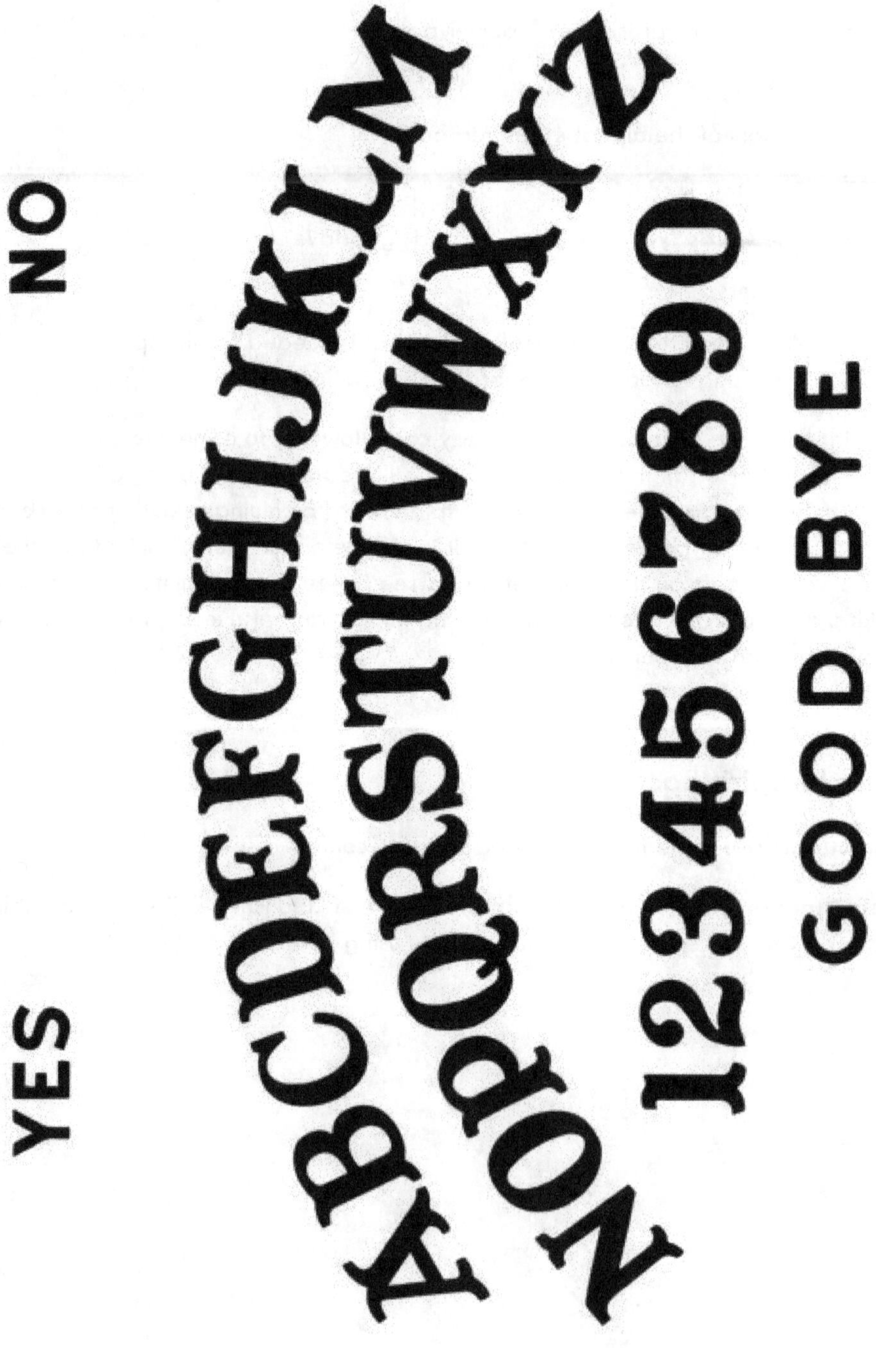
YES
NO
ABCDEFGHIJKLM
NOPQRSTUVWXYZ
1234567890
GOOD BYE

## Example Imaginal Exposure Script—*Self-Harm*

*I go into the bathroom and see a razor blade sitting on the bathroom counter. It was as if it were left out just for me. I barely hesitate and then use the blade to swiftly cut through the skin on my arm. I don't stop with one cut and continue onto my leg. Fresh blood pools at the surface. I knew the day would come where I would lose all control. Without even a knock, the bathroom door opens and my family is standing right in front of me. They scream and call 911. Shortly thereafter I hear the ambulances in the distance. The sounds get louder and louder until I am surrounded by officers and EMTs. I tell them my OCD took over and drove me to hurt myself. I am strapped into a stretcher and brought straight to the psychiatric unit. They tell me I will be there a long time with no visitors. They don't believe me that I was never trying to kill myself. I will be locked up forever and will never see my friends and family again.*

## Example Imaginal Exposure Script—*Hit and Run*

*I get into my car to drive to work on this rainy day. I buckle up and put on some music for my commute. I am driving along when I hear a scream and feel a bump underneath my tires. I think, Did I hit someone? I glance in the rearview mirror to see but there doesn't appear to be anything there. Then again, it is very foggy due to the rain so I can't be 100% sure. I have the urge to turn my around car to check, but I think it must all be in my head. When I get out of the car as I arrive at work, I see some red stains on my tires. I worry that it might be blood but try to reassure myself that I likely hit a dead animal that was already in the road. I head into work trying not to think about it. All of a sudden, the door to the office opens and several police officers are standing in front of me. They call me by name and tell me I am under arrest. They put me into the police car and drive me to the station, where I am then interrogated. The investigators tell me that I am in big trouble for leaving the scene of an accident. Tears are streaming down my face as they tell me I killed a pedestrian. My life is ruined and things will never be the same.*

## Example Imaginal Exposure Script—*Leaving the Stove On*

*I make some breakfast on the stove and get ready to leave. I am already running late. I usually check the stove to make sure it is turned off before I leave the house, but this time I forgot. I'm now too far from home to go back and check. I fear the house could be in flames but try to dismiss the thoughts as just an overactive imagination. Still, I can't shake the thought and try to call some friends and family members to check on the house while I am out just to make sure it is okay, but no one answers. My anxiety starts to rise and my heart is pounding. I hear my phone ring and I look down to see an unknown number. I pick up the call and it is the fire department in my town calling to notify me that there has been a fire in my home and to come back immediately. I jump into my car and drive home as fast as I can. Before I even turn onto my street, I can already see the smoke in the distance and smell the strong smell of fire. There are many firetrucks lined up on my street and firefighters working hard to put out the flames that are bursting out of the windows of my home. I pull over to the side of the road and get out of the car. I fall to the ground crying as I realize my pets are in the home as well as all of my treasured items. I am fully to blame and will never recover from this tragedy.*

# CHAPTER 9

# Acute Stress Disorder and Posttraumatic Stress Disorder

In this chapter, we will begin with a brief overview of the two primary disorders related to trauma, including discussions of diagnostic criteria and treatment considerations, and then provide exposures to help your clients who have trauma-related disorders face their fears. In addition, we will discuss safety behaviors to assess and eliminate for these disorders.

## WHAT ARE ACUTE STRESS DISORDER AND POSTTRAUMATIC STRESS DISORDER?

Acute stress disorder (ASD) and posttraumatic stress disorder (PTSD) are both psychiatric disorders entailing symptoms that emerge following a traumatic event. The main distinction between ASD and PTSD is the length of time the symptoms persist. ASD refers to acute trauma-related symptoms that last for less than one month following the traumatic event, whereas in PTSD, which often follows ASD, the symptoms have persisted for one month or more following the traumatic event (APA, 2013). Note that for either diagnosis to be made, the disturbance must cause significant distress or impairment in functioning and cannot be attributed to the effects of substance use or a medical condition or other mental disorder.

Both ASD and PTSD, according to the *DSM-5*, involve exposure to actual or threatened death, serious injury, or sexual violence. The individual either

1. directly experienced the event

2. witnessed the event happening to another person

3. heard of the event happening to a close family member or close friend, or

4. was exposed over and over to extremely horrific details of the event.

To diagnose ASD, the individual has to experience nine or more of the following symptoms for a period of three days to one month after being exposed to the traumatic event:

**Intrusive mental activity:**

- Recurrent, involuntary, intrusive, and distressing memories of the event

- Recurrent, distressing dreams that are related to the event

- Dissociative flashbacks in which it feels as if the event is happening again

- Intense or prolonged psychological distress or strong physiological reactions to cues that resemble the event

**Negative mood symptoms:**

- Persistent inability to experience positive emotions (e.g., happiness, satisfaction, love)

**Dissociative symptoms:**

- Altered sense of reality (e.g., "out of body experience," being in a daze, time slowing down)

- Inability to remember an important aspect of the event, not due to head injury, alcohol, or drugs

**Avoidant symptoms:**

- Efforts to avoid unpleasant memories, thoughts, or feelings related to the event

- Efforts to avoid external reminders (e.g., certain people, places, conversations, activities, objects, or situations) related to the event

**Symptoms of persistent hyperarousal:**

- Sleep disturbance (difficulty falling asleep, difficulty staying asleep, restless sleep)

- Irritable behavior and angry or aggressive outbursts, with little or no provocation

- Hypervigilance or excessive scanning of the environment for threat

- Difficulty concentrating

- Exaggerated startle response

As noted above, PTSD is diagnosed when a person experiences trauma-related symptoms lasting longer than one month following exposure to the trauma. Additionally, in PTSD, rather than experiencing any nine or more of the symptoms listed above, the individual must experience one or more intrusion symptom, one or both avoidance symptoms, two or more symptoms of negative change in cognition or mood, and two or more symptoms of altered arousal and activity, which can include reckless or self-destructive behavior.

An additional intrusive symptom often present in individuals with PTSD, but not ASD, is having strong physiological reactions to cues that resemble the traumatic event.

Additionally, several symptoms of negative change in cognition or mood can be present in PTSD but not ASD. These symptoms are as follows:

- Inability to remember an important aspect of the traumatic event, which is typically due to dissociative amnesia and not head injury or substance use

- Persistent and exaggerated negative belief or expectations about the self, others, or the world (e.g., "No one can be trusted"; "The world is dangerous.")

- Persistent distorted cognition about the cause or consequence of the traumatic event that leads to self-blame or placing blame on others

- Persistent negative emotional state, such as fear, horror, anger, guilt, or shame

- Significant decrease in interest or participation in significant activities

- Feeling detached or estranged from others

Epidemiologic research suggests that most adults have experienced, witnessed, or learned of a traumatic event in their lives (Breslau et al., 1998). Approximately 6% of adults and adolescents have a lifetime history of PTSD (Kessler et al., 2012). Some of the direct traumatic experiences that are often associated with PTSD include physical assault, sexual assault, serious accidents, combat, and natural disaster. For most people, traumatic experiences will not lead to the development or diagnosis of ASD, PTSD, or another prolonged psychiatric disturbance. It's important, therefore, not to assume someone has ASD or PTSD based on exposure to a traumatic experience alone. However, a subset of individuals who have experienced or witnessed a traumatic event will go on to develop a trauma-related disorder.

## Fear and Avoidance in Acute Stress Disorder/ Posttraumatic Stress Disorder

Fear and avoidance in ASD/PTSD can be of external or internal stimuli. Feared *external* stimuli may include situations or activities that appear "risky," such as driving on a highway or walking down a dark street. They may also include situations or activities that serve as reminders of the traumatic event; for example, a client with PTSD related to a motor vehicle accident might feel distressed and subsequently change the channel when an accident appears on TV, or may go to great lengths to avoid talking about the traumatic event. Feared *internal* stimuli include the traumatic memories themselves. People with ASD/PTSD often perceive their traumatic memories as threatening and might believe statements such as "If I allow myself to remember my trauma, I'll become so upset that I won't be able to handle it." When traumatic memories elicit fear, there is a natural tendency to try to suppress those thoughts by distracting oneself or using various "numbing" techniques. The problem is that suppression of thoughts tends to backfire, making those thoughts become even more intrusive and aversive (J. G. Beck, Gudmundsdottir, Palyo, Miller, & Grant, 2006; Wegner et al., 1987).

## Important Considerations in the Treatment of Acute Stress Disorder/Posttraumatic Stress Disorder

Though exposure-based therapy is efficacious for ASD (Bryant, Harvey, Dang, Sackville, & Basten, 1998), it is important to note that "critical incident stress debriefing" sessions—in which people (who often do not have ASD) are put into groups (often compulsorily) and asked to share traumatic memories—may do more harm than good (Rose, Bisson, Churchill, & Wessely, 2001; van Emmerik, Kamphuis, Hulsbosch, & Emmelkamp, 2002). Such sessions may disrupt the normal processing of trauma, "medicalize" normal trauma reactions and create an expectation of illness, and result in secondary traumatization (Bisson, 2003). We therefore caution that any early exposure-based interventions for trauma reactions be (a) completely voluntary, (b) done on an individual basis, and (c) limited to people with ASD.

Sometimes, PTSD occurs as a single diagnosis. However, comorbid anxiety disorders, depressive disorders, and substance use disorders are common and need to be taken into consideration. In some severe cases, particularly when recurrent trauma is experienced in childhood, the person experiences not only the symptoms of PTSD but also significant emotion regulation difficulties, disturbances in relational capacity, alterations in attention and consciousness (e.g., dissociation), adversely affected belief systems, and somatic distress or disorganization. Such cases have been called *complex PTSD* (Cloitre et al., 2009). Exposure can and should play a role in these clients' treatment as well, though they will often require some training in emotion regulation skills (e.g., Linehan, 2014) before launching into exposure.

# BEHAVIORAL TREATMENT FOR ACUTE STRESS DISORDER/POSTTRAUMATIC STRESS DISORDER

At the end of this chapter, we have included an imaginal exposure script for you to use with your client as a template. Your client can alter the script in order to individualize it since traumatic experiences are, in fact, so personal and specific to the event that occurred. For ease of use, we have categorized the exposure lists in this chapter based on five types of trauma:

1.  Posttraumatic fears related to physical assault

2.  Posttraumatic fears related to sexual assault

3.  Posttraumatic fears related to accidents

4.  Posttraumatic fears related to combat

5.  Posttraumatic fears related to disasters

## Posttraumatic Fears Related to Physical Assault

Physical (nonsexual) assault may take the form of muggings, beatings, shootings, stabbings, or threats of violence. PTSD stemming from physical attack is significantly more common in women, with 21% of women versus 2% of men who were physically attacked meeting criteria for PTSD (Kessler, Sonnega, Bromet, Hughes, & Nelson, 1995).

## Exposures for: Physical Assault-Related Fears

### In-Office Exposures: PHYSICAL ASSAULT-RELATED FEARS

- **Create an imaginal exposure script of the traumatic event.** Ask the client to write a narrative of the traumatic event. If the client cannot tell the entire story at once, writing down an aspect of it and reading it repeatedly can be a first step. You can also ask your client to record the narrative onto a smartphone or other recording device. When conducting imaginal exposure, we generally recommend encouraging the client to use present-tense language (e.g., "Now he is punching me" instead of "He punched me") and to include as much detail as possible, including what the client is seeing, hearing, smelling, feeling, tasting, and thinking. These procedures help the client access the cognitive and affective representations of the trauma memory, making the memory more vivid and the exposure more effective. (See the example script at the end of the chapter.)

- **Watch videos of physical assault.** Depending on the client's fears, this could start with online videos of boxing matches, progressing to street fighting and other forms of violence.

- **Look at pictures of injuries occurring to others.** With your client, conduct an online search for people who have been in a fight resulting in black eyes, missing teeth, or other injuries that might stem from being physically assaulted.

- **Listen to sounds of the traumatic experience.** Conduct an online search with your client of sounds related to the event that might be anxiety provoking. Then have the client repeatedly listen to the audio recordings of people crying, yelling, or screaming.

- **Look at pictures of the actual assault.** Have your client look at newspaper articles, mugshots of the perpetrator, or pictures of injuries from the client's assault if these are available.

## Out-of-Office Exposures: PHYSICAL ASSAULT-RELATED FEARS

- **Listen to the imaginal exposure recording.** Having already recorded a detailed narrative of the traumatic event in session, ask the client to listen to the recording on a daily basis at home. Have the client later listen to the recording while looking at pictures of assault or injury (either online or pictures of the actual assault).

- **Watch scary movies.** Ask your client to watch violent television shows or movies that the client has previously avoided.

- **Go into crowded places.** Have your client go to crowded places, such as to opening night of a big box office movie, to the theater, or to a sports event. This can be challenging because the client can't constantly scan for safety as there is so much going on in those venues.

- **Interact with "scary" people.** Here, the clinician and client must use their best judgment. Our aim is not to put the client in real danger. Rather, our goal is to have the client confront things that are scary, but not actually dangerous. We're not saying, therefore, that the client should walk through a bad part of town alone at night holding a wad of cash. But it may be possible to have the client interact with strangers or people who remind the client of the trauma. For example, if the client was assaulted by a tall man (and now fears tall men in general), it can be helpful to arrange experiences in which the client encounters other (safe) tall men.

## Safety Behaviors to Eliminate: PHYSICAL ASSAULT-RELATED FEARS

Some clients who have experienced physical assault will keep an exaggerated amount of distance between themselves and other people (e.g., remaining far enough that the other person cannot touch them). Encourage closer proximity to others.

## Posttraumatic Fears Related to Sexual Assault

Sexual assault, like all traumatic experiences, can occur in adulthood or in childhood. Among victims of adult rape, 46% of women and 65% of men meet criteria for PTSD. Among victims of child molestation, 25% of women and 12% of men meet criteria for PTSD (Kessler et al., 1995).

## Exposures for Sexual Assault-Related Fears

### In-Office Exposures: SEXUAL ASSAULT

- **Use imaginal exposure.** Ask the client to record a narrative of the traumatic event onto his smartphone or other recording device. For details, see "In-Office Exposures: Physical Assault-Related Fears" above. In cases of repeated sexual assault, start with a traumatic memory that the client perceives as aversive yet manageable; over time, work up to more strongly aversive memories.

- **Read accounts of sexual assault survivors.** Have your client go online and read first-hand accounts written by people who have survived sexual assault.

- **Lie on the ground.** You can ask your client if he is willing to lie down on the ground and then work up to having others hover over him.

## Out-of-Office Exposures: SEXUAL ASSAULT-RELATED FEARS

- **Listen to the imaginal exposure recording.** Having recorded a detailed narrative of the traumatic event in session, ask the client to listen to the recording on a daily basis at home.

- **Talk about the assault.** Your client might be ready to talk to others about the assault with family or trusted friends, or as part of a support group.

- **Watch movies or TV shows that include depictions of sexual assault.** Movies such as *The Prince of Tides, American History X, The Girl with the Dragon Tattoo,* and *I Spit on Your Grave* and TV shows such as *13 Reasons Why* (Season 1, episodes 9 and 12; Season 2, episode 13) have rape scenes of varying degrees of graphicness and brutality. Review these first before viewing them with the client.

- **Interact with "scary" people.** Again, our goal is never to create an objectively dangerous situation for the client. But we can identify whether the client is avoiding certain people, or certain kinds of people, who remind him of the trauma. For example, some sexual assault survivors might avoid men in general or people of the same age or race as their assailants. These would be viable targets for in vivo exposure.

- **Give or get hugs.** Your client may be willing to hug or get close to other people, such as friends or family members. Even if a friend or family member did not assault him, the client still may avoid getting close to any person. Have the client start by giving or receiving a quick hug and work up to a longer one.

- **For female clients: Resume yearly gynecological exams.** Following a sexual assault, your client may have stopped getting routine exams. If so, encourage her to resume this.

- **Go on a date.** If your client is single and has avoided dating for a long time, he can try going on a date. If the client is not ready to date, he can go on a dating website as an exposure to start talking with others who he may be interested in. This will help him get the ball rolling again with dating even if it does not lead to a date.

- **Visit the location of the assault.** Ask the client to visit the place where the sexual assault occurred, if possible.

## Safety Behaviors to Eliminate: SEXUAL ASSAULT-RELATED FEARS

PTSD is a significant risk factor for substance abuse, and clients with sexual assault trauma may be at particularly elevated risk. Encourage abstinence from substances during exposure therapy and consider augmenting exposure therapy with substance abuse treatment if necessary.

## Posttraumatic Fears Related to Accidents

Nine percent of women and 6% of men who have experienced a serious accident meet criteria for PTSD (Kessler et al., 1995). Here, we focus on motor vehicle accidents, which are the most common form of serious accident (Breslau et al., 1998). However, you can tailor these suggestions to fit the client's traumatic experience.

## Exposures for Accident-Related Fears

### In-Office Exposures: ACCIDENT-RELATED FEARS

- **Use imaginal exposure.** Ask the client to record a narrative of the traumatic event onto his smartphone or other recording device. For details, see "In-Office Exposures: Physical Assault-Related Fears" above.

- **Listen to audio clips of car crashes.** Do an online search with your client for "car brakes sound effects" to hear the sound of screeching brakes. Search for "car crash sound effects" to hear the sound of a collision.

- **Hold a mental image.** Ask your client to pick a "scene" from the accident and picture that scene with his eyes closed.

- **Read accounts of accidents.** Go online with your client and search for news stories about accidents that are similar to that experienced by the client.

- **Watch video clips.** Conduct online searches with your client for car accidents and watch videos of car crashes. Find the aspects of the video clips that are most anxiety provoking and have the client watch those repeatedly.

## Out-of-Office Exposures: ACCIDENT-RELATED FEARS

- **Listen to the imaginal exposure recording.** Having recorded a detailed narrative of the traumatic event in session, ask the client to listen to the recording on a daily basis at home.

- **Visit the accident location.** The client can visit the location of the accident and practice recalling the details of the event.

- **Drive.** Encourage the client to practice driving on his own, first in relatively low-threat situations such as quiet neighborhoods, then in higher-traffic areas or highways. Finally, the client should drive through the site of the accident repeatedly.

- **Drive with accident sounds playing.** The accident sounds described above (see "Listen to audio clips of car crashes") can be burned to a CD or loaded onto a smartphone. Have the client play them over and over again while driving—to the extent that it is objectively safe to do so.

- **Talk about the person who died.** If someone died during an accident, work with your client to talk about the person with others (either those who knew the deceased person or those who did not), look at pictures of the person, visit places that remind him of the person, or visit the person's grave.

## Safety Behaviors to Eliminate: ACCIDENT-RELATED FEARS

When clients with PTSD get back on the road, they may drive excessively slowly, sometimes even keeping their flashers on. In addition to being a safety behavior, this can also be dangerous. Encourage the client to keep up with traffic. Some clients will also "white-knuckle" the steering wheel as a means of increasing perceived control. Suggest a more relaxed grip.

Listening to the radio (thereby distracting oneself from anxiety) can serve as a safety behavior for some clients. In such cases, encourage driving in silence or with the exposure recording playing. On the other hand, for some clients, driving in a mildly distracted state (e.g., with the radio on) could be an exposure hierarchy item, in which case we *would* suggest having the radio on. Again, as is the case with many of the disorders reviewed in this book, the therapist's aim is to reverse the existing pattern of behavior: approach what is avoided, and stop what is comforting.

## Posttraumatic Fears Related to Combat

Among combat veterans, a staggering 39% meet criteria for PTSD (Kessler et al., 1995). To date, most of the epidemiologic research on combat-related PTSD has been in male veterans, though preliminary evidence suggests that combat-related PTSD is common in female veterans as well, perhaps even exceeding the risk in male veterans (Xue et al., 2015).

## Exposures for Combat-Related Fears

### In-Office Exposures: COMBAT-RELATED FEARS

- **Use imaginal exposure.** Ask the client to record a narrative of the traumatic event onto his smartphone or other recording device. For details, see "In-Office Exposures: Physical Assault-Related Fears" above. For many combat veterans, there will be several traumatic memories to consider. Start with a memory that the client perceives as aversive yet manageable; over time, work up to more strongly aversive memories.

- **Use virtual reality.** If you have VR equipment, the client can experience the sights by being able to look around in the virtually real world using the headset and hear sounds (e.g., helicopters, explosions) of a combat zone. The Virtually Better system, for example, has modules for Vietnam and Iraq/Afghanistan.

- **Listen to sounds of fireworks or explosions.** Do an online search for sounds of explosions or fireworks, especially bottle rockets, and listen to those repeatedly in the office together. Work toward listening to them with the volume increasingly louder.

- **Watch movie clips of combat.** Online, you can find combat scenes for your client to watch from movies such as *Saving Private Ryan, Platoon, American Sniper,* and *Black Hawk Down,* as well as several news clips showing combat in Iraq, Afghanistan, and elsewhere.

- **Sit with back to door.** Have your client sit in your office with his back to the door. Then have the client do this in other places in your office area, such as the waiting room, so that he can't scan the area as well (or at all).

## Out-of-Office Exposures: COMBAT-RELATED FEARS

- **Listen to the imaginal exposure recording.** Having recorded a detailed narrative of the traumatic event in session, ask the client to listen to the recording on a daily basis at home.

- **Sit in a crowded room.** Have your client go out to a movie theater or restaurant and choose a seat where he can't have his back to the wall. You can also ask your client to sit in the front of a room or the front of public transportation so that people are behind him.

- **Interact with "scary" people.** Some veterans feel fearful around people of the ethnic and racial backgrounds reminiscent of their traumatic experiences. Encourage the client to visit ethnic neighborhoods, shops, and restaurants and to interact with others there.

- **Attend a veteran's counseling group.** A veteran's counseling group is not only a helpful way to obtain much-needed social and emotional support, but it also can be a way for your client to begin talking about combat experiences.

- **See fireworks.** Ask the veteran to attend a fireworks show, such as on the 4th of July, in order to come in contact with the loud noises that resemble gunshots, as well as to be in crowded areas.

## Safety Behaviors to Eliminate: COMBAT-RELATED FEARS

Rates of substance abuse are high in veterans with PTSD, and use of substances (including alcohol and marijuana) may serve as a means of avoiding painful memories and emotions. Encourage the client to avoid the use of substances during exposure and consider referral for substance abuse treatment if indicated.

Some clients with combat-related PTSD will scan rooms, movie theaters, or restaurants while inside as a way to check that everything is safe. Encourage the client to try going out without scanning. This can include going for walks, going into stores, or sitting in restaurants.

## Posttraumatic Fears Related to Disasters

Five percent of women and 4% of men who are exposed to a disaster meet criteria for PTSD (Kessler et al., 1995). Fires, floods, earthquakes, and other natural disasters are all risk factors for the development of PTSD.

## Exposures for Disaster-Related Fears

### In-Office Exposures: DISASTER-RELATED FEARS

- **Use imaginal exposure.** Ask the client to record a narrative of the traumatic event onto his smartphone or other recording device. For details, see "In-Office Exposures: Physical Assault-Related Fears" above.

- **Read stories.** Conduct an online search with your client for natural disasters. If possible, see if you can find stories or articles related to the natural disaster your client experienced.

- **Watch movie clips of disasters.** The Internet offers a number of video clips of earthquakes, tornadoes, hurricanes, fires, and more to watch with your client in session. Focus on the parts of the clip that lead to the highest anxiety in your client and replay those parts repeatedly.

### Out-of-Office Exposures: DISASTER-RELATED FEARS

- **Listen to the imaginal exposure recording.** Having recorded a detailed narrative of the traumatic event in session, ask the client to listen to the recording on a daily basis at home.

- **Watch movies that include depictions of disasters.** Several movies, including *San Andreas, Twister, Backdraft,* and *The Day After Tomorrow* have realistic depictions of natural and human-made disasters. Have your client watch these movies at home.

## Safety Behaviors to Eliminate: DISASTER-RELATED FEARS

When watching a video clip or movie, your client might be distracted, peaking at it through his fingers, and so on. Ask the client to avoid using this safety behavior and instead to be fully engaged in the scenes. You can ask the client to fully describe the scene he is watching to prevent any subtle avoidance.

When writing the imaginal exposure script, some clients may want to hold back from putting in all of the gory details. Ask the client to make sure he has included all parts, including the most catastrophic thoughts, feelings, and scenes imaginable. You can go line by line over the story with your client and ask if any detail is missing that should be added to prevent the client from engaging in avoidance behavior.

As always, encourage the client to avoid the use of substances before or during exposure, and consider a referral for substance abuse treatment if indicated.

# CONCLUSIONS

PTSD and ASD are associated with two main categories of feared stimuli: external and internal. External feared stimuli can be situations or activities that are reminiscent of the traumatic event (e.g., news stories about assault), or they can be situations or activities that the client perceives as risky (e.g., driving at night). Internal feared stimuli are the traumatic memories themselves (e.g., one's memory of combat experiences) as well as the associated emotions. That is, people with PTSD and ASD perceive threats from both outside and inside themselves. In this chapter, we've provided you with some ideas about how to address both of these categories of fear, using in vivo exposure to feared external stimuli and detailed imaginal exposure to feared trauma memories. The aim, as with all exposure therapy, is to help the client recognize that these stimuli are not actually dangerous; in PTSD and ASD, we are also trying to help the client put the trauma into its proper perspective by disrupting vicious cycles of avoidance and thought suppression.

In the next chapter, we will discuss how to use exposure to treat clients with illness anxiety disorder. The chapter will provide various ideas for exposure for clients who avoid medical information as well as for those who tend to seek such information out.

# CHAPTER RESOURCES

**Reminder:** These resources are also available to download and print from http://www.newharbinger.com/43737.

### Example Imaginal Exposure Script—*Physical Assault*

*I am walking home from the store late at night when I hear footsteps coming closer to me. Without turning around, I quicken my pace and can see my car parked up ahead in the distance. Almost there. I reach into my pocket to grab my keys so that I can easily unlock my door, when all of a sudden I get hit from behind. I fall to the ground and can taste blood in my mouth. I see multiple pairs of shoes near my head, knowing that I am outnumbered. At least one person is holding me down while someone else is going through my pockets and belongings. I feel something cold pressed against my head and I fear it is a gun. I try not to move and tell them to take whatever they want. They tell me to shut up and I get kicked in my side as I yell in pain. I lose focus on the things around me and wonder when someone will come to help me. My eyes begin to close and I lose consciousness.*

### Example Imaginal Exposure Script—*Accident-Related PTSD*

*I'm driving home from work and it's raining heavily. I can barely see the road. I'm feeling nervous and I'm gripping the steering wheel. It feels like I'm going too fast, like the car is going to go out of control. I can just feel like something is about to happen. The cars are coming in the opposite direction, and I can see the glare of their headlights through the rain on my windshield. They seem like they're awfully close to me. I want to get off the road; I tell myself I shouldn't be driving in this weather. All of a sudden an oncoming car swerves into my lane and it all happens too fast for me to react. I hit the car head on and I can hear a sickening crunch of metal and the sound of breaking glass. I black out for a second, maybe longer, and when I come to, the airbag has deployed and I can't see anything in front of me. It's so hard to breathe. I can see that there's blood on the airbag and I realize that my nose is bleeding. My chest is throbbing from the seat belt and it feels like I broke a rib. My heart is going a mile a minute. I try to open the door but I can't budge it. As I try, I feel a stabbing pain in my wrist and in my head. I can barely see through the window, but I can see enough to know the driver of the other car appears to be in bad condition. I can see blood smeared across his window. I smell gasoline from the accident fill the air. It's strangely quiet and all I can hear is the sound of the rain falling on the roof of the car.*

## Example Imaginal Exposure Script—*Combat-Related PTSD*

*I am riding in the Humvee with three of my comrades. I am in full gear in 100 degree heat, sweating profusely, and my heart is pounding so loudly I am afraid even the enemy can hear it. Every bump in the road I fear could be an improvised explosive device. I've seen it happen too many times. Eventually we near our destination. All of a sudden there is a deafening explosion that rocks not only the vehicle but my entire body. My hearing is going out and I am disoriented. There is a piercing ringing. As the smoke clears, I look around to assess the scene and help those who may be wounded. Clutching my gun tightly, I go to my buddies. Some of them are still in the vehicle and are severely injured, while others are now on the side of the road, limp and bleeding profusely. I go to my best friend and hold him in my arms and tell him to hang on and make it until the medic arrives on scene. I can tell he is fading as his eyes begin to close. He dies in my arms. I hold him, looking around and wondering why this happened to him and not me. The guilt and sorrow I feel is unbearable.*

# CHAPTER 10

# Illness Anxiety Disorder

Illness anxiety disorder, derived from the older diagnosis of hypochondriasis, is a new diagnosis in the *DSM-5* (APA, 2013). This chapter will provide an overview of illness anxiety disorder and its treatment. In addition, we will provide detailed exposures to help your clients who have anxiety related to health conditions face their fears through in vivo, interoceptive, and imaginal exposure.

## WHAT IS ILLNESS ANXIETY DISORDER?

The *DSM-5* (APA, 2013) lists the criteria for illness anxiety disorder as:

A.  A preoccupation that one has, or will acquire, a serious disease.

B.  The person has no more than mild somatic symptoms. If a medical condition or risk of a medical condition is present, the person's preoccupation is clearly excessive to the actual illness or risk.

C.  The person is highly anxious about his or her health and is easily alarmed about his or her health status.

D.  Behavioral features can include excessive health-related behaviors *or* maladaptive avoidance.

E.  The anxiety is persistent (e.g., six months or more).

F.  The preoccupation is not better explained by another mental disorder.

The prevalence of illness anxiety disorder is not clear, in part because this diagnosis first appeared in the most recent *DSM* and therefore has not been the subject of major epidemiologic research. Estimates of the prevalence of hypochondriasis, the *DSM-IV* (APA, 2000) diagnosis from which the illness anxiety disorder diagnosis was partially derived, range from 0.2% (Looper & Kirmayer, 2001) to 5% (Faravelli et al., 1997).

## Fear and Avoidance in Illness Anxiety Disorder

In the diagnostic criteria, listed above, we see that illness anxiety disorder entails a fear of contracting a disease or having an underlying disease or condition that may have gone undiagnosed, despite repeated testing and frequent visits to primary care as well as specialists' offices. An individual with this fear will often be aware of any changes in bodily sensations and interpret these sensations as catastrophic in nature (e.g., slight tingling in an extremity means an onset of multiple sclerosis; a headache is interpreted as a brain aneurism, or a new mole or splotch on the arm is feared to be skin cancer). These bodily sensations or changes are not imagined and are, in fact, very real. It is therefore important to relay to your client that you understand that these symptoms are not "all in her head."

Individuals with illness anxiety will often seek repeated testing to ensure they are okay. Despite reassurance from doctors and negative tests results, an individual with these concerns may seek out confirmation from other doctors or go to specialists to continue to rule out a serious condition. These doctor visits and testing can become very costly as lab work, CT scans, X-rays, and MRIs are not inexpensive.

Conversely, some other clients with illness anxiety have an avoidant coping style, in which they avoid doctors' visits or other health-related information so that they do not receive "bad news" or are not reminded of their perceived illness or illness risk. Thus, there are two categories of behavioral dysfunction in illness anxiety: *information-seeking* and *information-avoidant*.

## Important Considerations in the Treatment of Illness Anxiety Disorder

The construct of illness anxiety disorder overlaps significantly with other anxiety-related disorders. Clients with panic disorder, for example, may also fear a medical catastrophe such as a heart attack. However, in panic disorder, these illness-related fears usually occur only when the client is having a panic attack, rather than being an ongoing concern. Clients with OCD may fear contracting a disease, usually via contamination. In illness anxiety disorder, on the other hand, the person tends to be preoccupied not with a concern about contracting a disease, but rather that she has a disease that has been undiagnosed or an underlying vulnerability to develop a disease.

The distinction between information-seeking and information-avoidant illness anxiety disorder is an important one because in exposure therapy, our aim is to *reverse the existing pattern of behavior*. That is, for information-seeking clients, we want them to stop their safety behaviors and tolerate the uncertainty of not knowing whether or not they have a disease. For information-avoiding clients, we want to expose them to information that they perceive as threatening.

The core fear of clients with illness anxiety may be death, but it may also be about being in pain, dealing with uncertainty, or seeing loved ones witness their deterioration. It is important to figure out your client's core fear so that you can target it directly in treatment.

# BEHAVIORAL TREATMENT FOR ILLNESS ANXIETY DISORDER

In addition to providing exposures that can be applied broadly to clients with illness anxiety disorder, we have also, where appropriate, listed specific exposures that can be used for clients with the following common concerns:

**Cardiac**—Individuals with illness anxiety may have concerns about having a heart attack or underlying heart disease. They may monitor their blood pressure, be overly cautious about engaging in physical activity, and make excessive trips to the doctor.

**Cancer/Tumors**—Cancer is another common concern among individuals with illness anxiety. This fear may include having cancer that has gone undiagnosed and is getting worse. It can include any type of cancer, including breast cancer, a tumor, or skin cancer. Information-seeking clients may excessively check their skin or feel for spots in the body, such as by doing breast self-exams. Conversely, information-avoidant clients might avoid checking themselves or getting any kind of screening at all.

**HIV/AIDS**—Having undiagnosed HIV/AIDS can be a concern for those with illness anxiety. A client with this fear may avoid intimacy with others or may be overly cautious (e.g., going to get HIV testing regularly).

**Degenerative neurological disorders**—Degenerative neurological disorders, such as multiple sclerosis (MS) or amyotrophic lateral sclerosis (ALS), can be cause for concern for those who have illness anxiety. Individuals with this fear may be concerned about muscle twitching in the extremities, weakness in an area of the body, or changes in vision.

**Insanity**—Individuals with illness anxiety may fear having a serious mental health condition. For example, a client with this fear may be concerned about losing her mind or developing a severe mental disorder, and thus potentially being thrown into an "insane asylum." Many movies depict frightening scenes of being locked up in a padded cell, and these kinds of images may come to mind when one is concerned with becoming mentally ill.

Remember, our general strategy is to reverse the existing pattern of behavior. So for information-avoidant clients, we want to lead them to more and more "scary" information. For information-seeking clients, we want them to put the brakes on their safety behaviors. This distinction is important as you do not want to assign an exposure of going to the doctor for a check-up to an information-seeking client, for example.

Although illness anxiety disorder is diagnostically distinct from panic disorder, in both conditions, as noted above, clients can fear catastrophic illness (e.g., a heart attack or stroke). Interoceptive exposure, therefore, can be useful in the treatment of both disorders. We have included exposures to help target these fears; however, we also encourage you to reference chapter 6 on panic disorder for a more exhaustive list that outlines additional interoceptive ideas for clients.

Included at the end of the chapter are a variety of imaginal exposure scripts for specific concerns related to illness anxiety. Use these with your client as a template, adding to and adjusting them to make the script more individualized to the client. Just as in chapter 6, which contains a sample letter to send to the client's physician to obtain confirmation that interoceptive exposures are safe for the client, we encourage you to be in contact with the physician prior to beginning the interoceptive illness anxiety exposures as well.

# Exposures for Illness Anxiety

## In-Office Exposures: ILLNESS ANXIETY

- **Conduct interoceptive exposures.** Because people with illness anxiety disorder often fear catastrophic medical events, we recommend that you and the client practice facing the bodily sensations that elicit fear. Below are some examples of interoceptive exposures for various types of health concerns:
  - **Cardiac concerns:** Have the client run in place, walk quickly, go to the gym, drink caffeine, and do what she can to get her heart rate up. Ask your client to drink espresso or an energy drink, which may lead to a racing heart. Refer to chapter 6 for additional ideas to get the heart racing or pounding.
  - **Degenerative neurological disorders (e.g., MS, ALS):** Exercises such as hyperventilation and keeping the arms raised can lead to tingling sensations, which may trigger fears of a degenerative neurological illness.
  - **Insanity:** Exercises that induce depersonalization or derealization can be used, such as staring at oneself in a mirror, being in a room with a strobe light, or staring at light coming through a venetian blind. We also recommend having the client spin in place while standing or sitting in a chair with wheels to feel disoriented.

- **Read scary stories.** Do online searches with your client to find stories about people who have experienced or died from the feared medical condition. Ask your client to repeatedly re-read the parts of the story that evoke the most anxiety.

- **Say scary phrases.** Have your client repeat feared phrases such as "I have a brain tumor," "I have AIDS," "I am going insane," and so on.

- **Create an imaginal exposure script.** Create a detailed script about experiencing, and even dying from, the feared medical condition. (See the imaginal exposure scripts at end of this chapter.)

- **Get "bad" news.** Practice giving the client bad medical news. Review with the client beforehand the fact that you're planning to give her bad news—we're not looking to fool the client. Some examples include:
  - **Cardiac concerns:** Set up an exposure with your client in which you measure her blood pressure or heart rate in session and tell her that it is abnormally high and, therefore, very concerning.
  - **Cancer/Tumors:** Role-play giving your client the bad news that she has stage 4 cancer.
  - **HIV/AIDS:** Role-play giving your client the news that she has now been diagnosed with AIDS and has X amount of years to live.

- **Degenerative neurological disorders**: Make a list of symptoms of your client's feared disorders and print it out. Look at the paper seriously and then say, "You do appear to have multiple sclerosis, as you have most of the symptoms needed for diagnosis."

- **Insanity**: Tell the client, "It is my opinion that you are clinically insane." Remember, this needs to be planned out and conducted collaboratively with the client. We're not looking to fool her; we just want the client to practice hearing the scary words.

- **Write a self-obituary.** Ask your client to write her own obituary, indicating that she died from the feared illness. You can then read the obituary to the client and also ask her to read it aloud. To make the exposure more intense, ask the client to read it (or listen as you read it aloud) while looking at pictures of coffins, cemeteries, or funeral processions.

## Out-of-Office Exposures: ILLNESS ANXIETY

- **Conduct interoceptive exposures.** These interoceptive exposures can be conducted out of the office:

  - **Cardiac concerns**: Ask your client to go to a steam room or other area that might make her experience feared sensations such as feeling hot or sweaty. When appropriate and not dangerous to do so, your client can sit in the car on a summer day with the windows rolled up for a few minutes to try to create the feared sensation of being overheated and having a racing heart due to the hot conditions.

  - **Degenerative neurological disorders (e.g., MS, ALS)**: Interoceptive exposures that elicit a tingling sensation in the extremities can be helpful, including hyperventilating or keeping the arms elevated.

  - **Insanity**: The client can do exercises that induce depersonalization or derealization, such as staring at oneself in a mirror, being in a room with a strobe light, or staring at light coming through a venetian blind. The client should practice doing this while out of the office, such as in the parking lot of a state hospital or while home alone and watching a movie about mental illness, to make it more anxiety provoking.

- **Watch movies.** Ask your client to watch online video clips, movies, or television shows related to the feared medical condition. Watching it while home alone will make it even more challenging. Have your client pay special attention to the parts of the movie that create the most anxiety and replay those parts repeatedly. Some movies that might be effective include:

  - **Cardiac concerns**: *The Widowmaker*

  - **Cancer/Tumors**: *A Walk to Remember, The Fault in Our Stars, Dying Young, Terms of Endearment,* and *Stepmom*

- **HIV/AIDS**: *Philadelphia, Rent, The Normal Heart,* and *The Hours*
- **Degenerative neurological disorders (e.g., MS, ALS):** *The Theory of Everything, Gleason,* and *I Am Breathing*
- **Insanity:** *A Beautiful Mind, Split, Shutter Island, One Flew Over the Cuckoo's Nest,* and *Girl, Interrupted*

- **Read obituaries.** Have your client read obituaries while at home, as she may come across some stories in the newspaper or online about someone who died from the feared medical condition.

- **Visit a cemetery.** Go with your client to a cemetery or ask her to do this outside of the session if she has fears about death related to a medical illness. First, have your client practice driving by the cemetery, then work toward driving through the cemetery, getting out of the car, and then later walking around and looking at headstones. You can have your client bring along the imaginal exposure script she wrote and read it while sitting in the cemetery.

- **Pretend to have the feared illness.** Strategies to have your client pretend to be sick in your office include:
  - **Cardiac concerns:** Encourage the client to clutch her chest or slur her words, to mimic signs of a heart attack or stroke.
  - **Cancer/Tumors:** The client can wear a head scarf, as is often worn by chemotherapy patients to conceal hair loss.
  - **Insanity:** Purchase a straitjacket costume (often sold for Halloween) from an online retailer and have the client wear it in session. To make the exposure more challenging, you can ask your client to wear it while she listens to a recording of the imaginal exposure script or while watching a movie of someone who has been institutionalized due to severe mental illness. Alternatively, have your client go to a store or other public area and talk to herself aloud.

- **Visit the hospital or volunteer.** The client can volunteer to help others with the feared medical condition. Generally, this would require your client to register as a volunteer with the hospital. Alternatively, it might be helpful (assuming you have adequate permission) for your client to simply sit in the waiting room of a medical unit specializing in the feared illness (e.g., a cardiac clinic, an oncology unit).

- **Get avoided medical tests.** Information-avoidant clients will often avoid needed medical tests for fear of getting bad news. Therefore, encourage these clients to obtain tests, as shown for specific concerns below:
  - **Cardiac concerns:** Clients can ask their physician to check their blood pressure or administer an EKG.
  - **Cancer/Tumors:** Clients can visit a dermatologist to get checked for skin cancer.
  - **HIV/AIDS:** Clients can visit their physician or a reproductive health clinic to be tested for HIV and other sexually transmitted diseases.

## Safety Behaviors to Eliminate: ILLNESS ANXIETY

Many clients will avoid any activity that may change their bodily sensations (e.g., racing or pounding heart), such as exercise, sex, or caffeine. Therefore, make sure that these activities are reintroduced as soon as possible. Some clients say they used to love to drink coffee but gave it up to prevent anxiety. Help the client get back to the previous routines before anxiety became so prominent.

Clients with illness anxiety may seek reassurance from family members, friends, or doctors. Ask your client to refrain from seeking reassurance from others. In addition, if you meet with friends and family members, you can have them answer the question that the client poses to them once and then each time after that say, "I already told you what I thought, and I am not going to tell you again as I do not want to make your anxiety worse in the long run." Later on (and with the client's permission), you can have the family member refrain from giving reassurance altogether and then (even more challenging) say the opposite of what the client wants to hear. For example, if the client asks a family member, "Do you think my heart racing is a sign of heart attack?" the family member could say, "Yes, it very well might be a heart attack."

Many information-seeking individuals with illness anxiety will report spending a lot of time conducting online searches of symptoms in an attempt to reassure themselves that they are not at risk. This should be eliminated early in therapy. You can set up some structure as to how to limit the searching online. For example, if you have a client who is spending two hours per day on the Internet checking and researching symptoms, it may not be feasible right away to tell them to stop altogether. Therefore, work with the client to add items to the hierarchy that include spending less than an hour per day research-ing symptoms on the Internet, going one day without conducting any online searches of symptoms, spending only thirty minutes four times a week researching symptoms, and so on, until the problematic behavior has stopped.

Clients with information-seeking illness anxiety may repeatedly check themselves for signs of illness. For example, clients with cardiac illness might check their blood pressure or heart rate at home using a monitor, or simply check their pulse with their fingertips. Those with cancer-related concerns might engage in repetitive body checking and scan-ning for lumps, bumps, or discoloration of the skin. Clients with HIV fears may get tested repeatedly and unnecessarily. Talk to your client about eliminating these behaviors.

In contrast, clients with the information-avoidant type of illness anxiety may distract themselves from really thinking about their symptoms by trying to keep busy or by changing the topic of conversation if it is anxiety-provoking. Ask the client to refrain from distraction, stay engaged in the conversation, and pay attention to the symptoms rather than avoiding them. Some clients may have asked other people in their lives to not talk about certain anxiety-provoking topics; encourage the client to let people talk about whatever they want to talk about without being afraid of upsetting the client.

# CONCLUSIONS

Illness anxiety disorder can be a debilitating condition. Individuals often present with high levels of anxiety as well as avoidance or checking behaviors in an effort to alleviate the intense anxiety about having a medical condition that could have gone undetected. We have highlighted major categories of concerns that are frequently seen among those with illness anxiety, including cardiac concerns, cancer, HIV/AIDS, degenerative neurological disorders, and a concern about going "crazy." You can use these exposures as they are written and can also individualize them to fit the needs of the specific concerns of your client, which will lead to the most optimal outcomes.

In the next and last chapter, we will introduce you to ways in which you can help both adults and children who have separation anxiety. We will provide many exposure ideas for you to use with your client to target a fear of being separated from an attachment figure.

# CHAPTER RESOURCES

### Example Imaginal Exposure Script—*Cardiac Concerns*

*I have been feeling slight pains on the left side of my chest. My doctor has told me that everything is fine and not to worry…it's only anxiety. I'm not so sure and feel that my doctors are incompetent and that something is terribly wrong. They tend to think it is only in my head and I am just being dramatic. I try to stay calm. All of a sudden, the pains in my chest worsen and I grab my chest and fall to the hard, wooden floor. My mind is racing and I think, I knew I should have never listened to my doctors. My breathing quickens and I begin to feel dizzy. Things seem unreal around me. My phone is out of reach and there is no one around to save me. This is it. I'm about to die. I should have never listened to my doctors.*

### Example Imaginal Exposure Script—*Cancer*

*This is what my life has become. I am hooked up to machines and being fed poison to fight the poison that has already made a home for itself in my body. This cancer has consumed my entire life. I am either sitting in a doctor's office, talking on the phone with a doctor, reading about cancer, talking about it with friends and family, or trying to comfort those around me who are most scared by my diagnosis. Having beautiful hair is a thing of my past. I have watched it come out chunk by chunk and be littered across my house before I made the painful decision to shave the rest of it off. While I spend most of my days feeling ill, unable to eat much, and remembering the life I once had, I am most scared of what lies ahead. I am full of fear and anxiety. The doctors say, "Take one day at a time," but even that sounds incredibly overwhelming. I can't stand this anymore. I am no longer my own person and have so little dignity left.*

## Example Imaginal Exposure Script—*AIDS*

*For the past year I've had so many unexplained medical symptoms, such as weight loss, fatigue, and these weird splotches on my skin. I have always avoided the doctor because it causes me so much anxiety, but I finally decided to go get checked out at the urging of my family. During the exam, my doctor tells me he recommends I get tested for HIV/AIDS. Immediately I am filled with terror and flash back to all of the times I could have come into contact with the virus. I agree to the testing but do so reluctantly. My palms are sweaty and my heart is racing as I face into my fear and pray that this will probably be fine in the end.*

*In the days to come, I wait and wait for my test results, constantly checking my voicemail to hear from the doctor. No news. Eventually I think, No news must be good news. As time goes by, I almost forget about the results until I pick up my cell phone one afternoon. My doctor tells me, "I'm sorry. You have AIDS." He starts to tell me the next steps but I hear nothing. I am frozen in time. The room spins and I cannot focus. How did I get this and who did I infect? I hear the doctor tell me how advanced the disease is and how I don't have much time left. I should have been tested sooner.*

## Example Imaginal Exposure Script—*Going Insane*

*I open my eyes and the room is unfamiliar. It is cold and dark and small. I start to come to and realize I am in a padded cell. I can't move my arms. I can't move my feet. I struggle to see what is holding me down, only to see metal clamps keeping my limbs planted firmly to this bed. I start to call out, "Hello?" No one answers. I panic and begin to yell, "Get me outta here!!!!" I struggle to get free but there is no hope. I hear a voice talking to me, telling me that the government is who did this to me. I knew they were bad. They've been after me all these years, watching me through my window, following me to the grocery store, calling my phone pretending to me telemarketers. I knew they were watching me and now here I am.*

*A man dressed in white enters the room with a tray of medications and a small glass of water. I know they want me to swallow a tracking device masqueraded as a pill so that they can watch all my moves. I refuse to open my mouth, but the man is stronger than me and I have to take it. He tells me, "It's okay; the medicine will help you feel better and you will feel more like yourself. You've had a psychotic episode." I have flashes of my "old" self working, taking care of my family, and having fun in my life. I vaguely remember how I slowly started to feel like things were "off" with me and I started hearing sounds when no sounds were there. I feared losing my mind but dismissed the thoughts. I should have trusted myself back then and looked for help because this is my new home now.*

# CHAPTER 11

# Separation Anxiety Disorder

This chapter will cover the definition of separation anxiety disorder and how it manifests differently in children and adults. We provide some important treatment considerations and discuss how separation anxiety in children and adolescents may result in school refusal. This chapter will include various types of exposures for children, adolescents, and adults with the disorder.

## WHAT IS SEPARATION ANXIETY DISORDER?

Nearly 7% of adults and adolescents have a lifetime history of separation anxiety disorder (Kessler et al., 2012), a condition that is most commonly seen in children but which can be present in adults as well. The *DSM-5* (APA, 2013) outlines the criteria for separation anxiety disorder as follows:

A. An excessive and developmentally inappropriate fear about separation from an attachment figure, with at least three of the following symptoms:

1. Excessive distress about separating from home or attachment figures

2. Excessive worrying about losing attachment figures or about harm coming to them

3. Excessive worrying about experiencing an event, such as getting lost, that would result in separation from an attachment figure

4. Reluctance to go away from home, to school, or to other places due to fears of separation from an attachment figure

5. Fear of being alone or without an attachment figure

6. Reluctance to sleep without being near an attachment figure

7. Nightmares about separation

8. Physical symptoms (e.g., headaches, stomachaches) in response to actual or anticipated separation from an attachment figure

B. The fear and avoidance are persistent (e.g., four weeks in children, six months in adults).

C.  The fear and avoidance cause significant distress or functional impairment.

D.  The fear and avoidance cannot be better explained by another mental health disorder, such as agoraphobia, psychotic disorders, or autism spectrum disorder.

## Fear and Avoidance in Separation Anxiety Disorder

Individuals with separation anxiety disorder fear being separated from a major attachment figure, such as a parent or spouse. Thus, daily activities such as going to school or work can be frightening. Fears in separation anxiety disorder may be expressed as somatic symptoms or as nightmares. The hallmark cognitive feature of separation anxiety disorder is worrying about catastrophes. Specifically, clients with this disorder may worry excessively about something bad happening to an attachment figure—for example, that a parent will become ill, get injured, or die. They may also worry that something will happen that will cause separation from the figure—for example, that they will get lost or be kidnapped.

Children with separation anxiety disorder may refuse to attend school or other activities outside of the home or away from parents. Adults with separation anxiety disorder may be unable to attend work or even leave the home without a trusted attachment figure. Clients with separation anxiety may also have difficulty being home alone, or going to sleep alone, without the attachment figure present.

## Important Considerations in the Treatment of Separation Anxiety Disorder

Some anxiety related to separation from a caregiver at a young age, such as in a toddler, is very common and is part of a normal phase of development. However, as the individual becomes older, it may be indicative of an anxiety disorder. It is important to determine the developmental appropriateness of the fear and avoidance before diagnosing separation anxiety disorder.

Note that there is a behavioral overlap with agoraphobia; in both conditions, the person may be reluctant to go places, or be home alone, without a trusted other person. The critical difference is that in agoraphobia, the individual primarily fears experiencing panic-like symptoms or their consequences, whereas in separation anxiety disorder the person primarily fears separation from the attachment figure. It is therefore critical to assess the core fears for an accurate differential diagnosis. For a discussion of exposure for agoraphobia, please see chapter 6.

# BEHAVIORAL TREATMENT FOR SEPARATION ANXIETY DISORDER

We have divided this chapter into exposures for children and exposures for adults, as this disorder may manifest differently in these two age groups. We have also included a section specifically targeted for clients who refuse to go to school, although school refusal is not exclusive to separation anxiety (that is, kids with a wide range of anxiety-related disorders might refuse to attend school). If your client refuses to attend school, addressing this will be a major component of the treatment, with the goal of helping the child or adolescent return to school as soon as possible. We will provide exposure ideas for how to help your younger client resume routine schooling.

## Behavioral Treatment for Children and Adolescents with Separation Anxiety Disorder

When conducting exposures with a child or adolescent who has separation anxiety, keep in mind the appropriateness of exposures based on the developmental level of the client. For example, it would not be appropriate to leave a seven-year-old child with separation anxiety home alone for several hours with no supervision. Therefore, the exposures listed below will need to be tailored to the client's age.

We recommend that you refer to chapter 4, which focuses on how to help younger clients with anxiety. This is often a good time to use rewards for the child's brave behavior when doing exposures.

# Exposures for Children and Adolescents
## with Separation Anxiety

In-Office Exposures: **CHILDREN AND ADOLESCENTS WITH SEPARATION ANXIETY**

- **Create distance.** Have your client practice being separated from his attachment figure while in your office for a session. You may need to start with your office door open and the attachment figure sitting in the hallway. You can then advance to shutting the office door with the younger client knowing that his attachment figure is directly outside the door. Slowly create more and more distance from the attachment figure in each session to the point where the client's attachment figure might stay in the car for a session and will eventually drop the client off and run an errand.

- **Create an imaginal exposure script.** Create a detailed story with the client about his worst fears about separating from his parent, caregiver, or other attachment figure. (See the imaginal exposure script at the end of this chapter.)

- **Play a game.** Play a game with your client in which you go back and forth coming up with all the scary things that could be happening to the attachment figure at that very moment while the client is in your office. See who can "win" the game by coming up with most ideas (e.g., attachment figure getting struck by lightning, getting into a car accident when going out for coffee while the child is in session, having a heart attack in the waiting room).

- **No goodbyes.** Instruct the attachment figure to drive away from the session for a few minutes without the child's saying "Goodbye;" "I love you;" or anything else comforting. You can later have the child work toward saying things such as "Don't drive safely" or "I hope you get into an accident" to the attachment figure before they separate from each other.

## Out-of-Office Exposures: CHILDREN AND ADOLESCENTS WITH SEPARATION ANXIETY

- **Be on different floors of the home.** Ask the child to spend time on the second floor of the house while the attachment figure is on the first floor of the house or in the basement. Slowly increase the time spent on different floors of the home.

- **Take a walk or bike ride.** Ask the child to take a walk or ride his bike away from home for one minute and then slowly increase the amount of time spent away from the home.

- **Get a babysitter.** Ask the attachment figure to go out for a short period of time (e.g., thirty minutes) and have a babysitter stay home with the child. When this gets easier for the child, the parents can go out for longer periods of time.

- **Be separated for an undetermined amount of time.** Set up an exposure in which the attachment figure tells the child he or she is running an errand and doesn't know how long it will take. This is helpful in challenging the child to manage more ambiguous situations in which he does not have all the details. You can tell the attachment figure to make the exposure brief (ten to fifteen minutes), but the child will not have this information.

- **Go to a sleepover.** Ask the child to make plans to go to a sleepover. To make the exposure more challenging, you can assess what factors would make this exposure more difficult, such as whether or not the child is staying over at a friend's or family member's house or how far the child will be from home. Modify these variables as appropriate to change the level of difficulty of the exposure.

- **Attend a camp.** Work toward having your client go to a day camp during the summer or eventually a sleepaway camp, especially if it is something he might have wanted to do if anxiety didn't interfere with that desire.

## Safety Behaviors to Eliminate: CHILDREN AND ADOLESCENTS WITH SEPARATION ANXIETY

Often children or adolescents will seek reassurance from the "safety person" (see chapter 6) that he or she will be okay. Try to eliminate this reassurance. Eventually, the attachment figure should be instructed to say things like "I don't know if I will be okay," or "No, something bad may happen while I am out of the house." The child should be told when this safety behavior is going to be eliminated and when the attachment figure is going to start saying the opposite of what the child (or child's anxiety) wants to hear.

Children and adolescents may end up using applications on their cell phones to locate where the attachment figure is at all times (through a GPS). First, limit the use of these apps (e.g., starting with reduced checking time) and then work toward deleting the apps altogether. If the child finds it too challenging to delete the app, the attachment figure can turn off his or her GPS location so that the child can't access it.

Ask the child to reduce clinginess or hanging on to the parent or other attachment figure. Also work with your client to reduce the number of times he is calling or texting to check in with the attachment figure, such as when home with a babysitter or in another location away from the attachment figure.

## Behavioral Treatment for School Refusal

School refusal, while not a DSM-5 diagnosis, can create significant distress for the client, family members, and school personnel. School refusal is not only a consequence of separation anxiety disorder but can also be related to panic, social anxiety, depression, or other concerns. It is beyond the scope of this book to outline all of the treatment interventions for school refusal, though behavioral interventions are often a major aspect of treatment. We have included exposure ideas for helping the child or adolescent return to school while you continue to work with him on the reasons for school avoidance, such as separation anxiety disorder, social anxiety, or another anxiety-related disorder. Note that most of the exposure exercises for school refusal are out-of-office exposures, as the child must gradually take steps to be in school.

There are books devoted to in-depth protocols for the treatment of school refusal. We have included the exposure component of the treatment here, but we note that other interventions are often needed for a more thorough and complete treatment. School refusal treatment should also involve parents, teachers, and staff at the school as well as a specific reentry plan.

# Exposures for School Refusal

## In-Office Exposures: SCHOOL REFUSAL

- **Interoceptive exposures.** For the child who refuses to go to school due to fears of having panic-like sensations, practice doing interoceptive exposures to address feared bodily sensations that occur—or that the child fears will occur—while at school, such as dizziness or shortness of breath. As described in chapter 6, interoceptive exposures can include strategies to:
  - Induce feelings of heat flashes, such as wearing warm clothing
  - Induce lightheadedness, such as hyperventilating or getting up quickly
  - Induce shortness of breath, such as breathing through a straw
  - Induce dizziness, such as spinning in a chair
  - Increase heart rate, such as running in place
  - Induce mild derealization, such as staring at lights or spinning circles online

- **Role-plays for social anxiety.** For the child who refuses to go to school because of fears of interpersonal interactions, role-play these challenging interactions (with confederates if possible), providing feedback as you go. You can find a long list of these role-play exposures in chapter 7. Briefly, in-office exposures for socially anxious children can include:
  - Practicing giving class presentations or speaking up in class
  - Practicing using a public restroom
  - Practicing starting and maintaining conversations, including making small mistakes on purpose
  - Getting comfortable with embarrassment by doing "silly" things in front of confederates or deliberately looking anxious in front of others

- **Role-plays for returning to school.** It may also be useful to give particular attention to role-playing conversations about the child's (sometimes prolonged) absence from school. When a child returns to school after an absence, it's not unusual for peers to ask where he has been. Children with school refusal often find this conversation uncomfortable, thus leading to more avoidance. We often encourage a "little white lie" here, in which the child explains that he had an illness or injury, and then shifts the topic to ask his peers what he missed.

## Out-of-Office Exposures: SCHOOL REFUSAL

- **Ride the school bus.** If the child is used to having his attachment figure drive him to school and engage in lengthy goodbyes, it may be helpful to work toward having the child start taking the bus to school.

- **Take a walk.** Ask the younger client to go to the school during school hours but only to walk around the building a few times without entering it.

- **Eat in the cafeteria.** If the child has not been to school, consider asking the child to go to school only for lunchtime, which can be less stressful for the client but will help him get back into the school building during school hours.

- **Go to recess.** Encourage the client to return to school only for recess time. Once the child has demonstrated that he can stay at school for the entirety of recess, then add on time that the child is in school before and after recess time.

## Safety Behaviors to Eliminate: SCHOOL REFUSAL

Work with your client to reduce the number of times he is calling or texting to check in with the attachment figure when at school.

# Behavioral Treatment for Adults with Separation Anxiety Disorder

Though separation anxiety disorder is more commonly seen in children, it can present in adults as well. As discussed above, a careful differential diagnosis is required to distinguish separation anxiety disorder from agoraphobia, in which the client may feel a need to have a trusted companion in situations in which escape would be difficult or in which it would be difficult to get help.

## Exposures for Adults with Separation Anxiety

### In-Office Exposures: ADULTS WITH SEPARATION ANXIETY

- **Create an imaginal exposure script.** Create a detailed imaginal exposure script with your client about his feared outcome when separated from a spouse, parent, or other figure.

- **Say scary phrases.** Ask your client to repeat feared phrases such as "My husband is going to die when coming home from work today." Increase the difficulty of this exposure by having the client say this phrase while looking at pictures of his spouse.

- **Read an online article.** Do an online search with your client to find articles describing situations that are similar to his fears, such as people whose spouses have been killed in accidents, people who have been attacked or mugged, and so on.

- **Watch online video clips.** Find video clips online of individuals who were injured, attacked, or died when alone. Watch these clips repeatedly with the client and have the client repeat phrases such as "This could happen to me" or "This could happen to my wife."

## Out-of-Office Exposures: ADULTS WITH SEPARATION ANXIETY

- **Create more distance.** Ask your client to start increasing the time spent away from his attachment figure. For example, if the client will not run errands without the attachment figure, have him start planning small trips to the bank, and then the grocery store, and then plan other activities that increase the amount of time separated from the person on purpose (e.g., not just due to being at work).

## Safety Behaviors to Eliminate: ADULTS WITH SEPARATION ANXIETY

Adults with separation anxiety may seek reassurance from the attachment figure that he or she will be okay. Encourage the client to discontinue this behavior, and coach the attachment figure to decline to answer the questions should they come up.

Remove applications on the client's cell phone that enable the client to locate where the attachment figure is at all times (through a GPS). Also work with your client to reduce the number of times he is calling or texting to check in with the attachment figure.

# CONCLUSIONS

Separation anxiety can be debilitating and can negatively interfere with the lives of both children and adults. Separation anxiety in children and adolescents can result in a refusal to attend school. However, it is important to note that school refusal can be related to other psychological disorders as well, such as depression or social anxiety. Individuals with separation anxiety may also have difficulty being home alone or separated in any way from the attachment figure. The exposure ideas included in this chapter will be helpful in allowing individuals with separation anxiety to face their fears and resume normal activity.

# CHAPTER RESOURCES

**Reminder:** These resources are also available to download and print from http://www.newharbinger.com/43737.

### Example Imaginal Exposure Script—*Separation Anxiety Disorder*

*I am getting ready for my sleepover at a friend's house and I start getting a pit in the bottom of my stomach. My heart starts racing and I worry about being away from my parents. I hate sleeping away from home and worry something really bad could happen to my mom and dad. My parents tell me I have to go. I get in the car and start to cry. My mind starts creating scary images of my parents getting sick, getting into a car accident, or even dying. Something bad will happen if I am not with them. I make it to the sleepover and have fun until it's time to go to bed. I lie awake waiting for something bad to happen and try to count down the minutes until I am home. My anxiety then gets worse and worse and I feel like I can barely breathe. I call my mom's cell phone and there is no answer. I call my dad's cell phone next and there is no answer. I then frantically start dialing our house phone to see if either of them will pick up the phone. No answer. I see police lights in the distance lighting up the dark night. They are coming closer and closer to where I am staying. I am about to receive some really bad news.*

## Let's Separate Game!

**Materials:**

- Prewritten or blank template provided below

- Pen or pencil

- Scissors

**Rules:** Cut up the prewritten template provided below, and divide the pieces of paper into three piles: (1) amount of time the attachment figure will spend separated from the child, (2) where the attachment figure will go, and (3) what the therapist and child will say repeatedly in the office during the exposure. In addition to the prewritten template, we have included a blank template on which you can customize the times, places, and things to say to suit the needs of the client. For each round, the child will blindly choose a piece of paper from each pile, thus creating the framework for the exposure. Set the timer and get separating! Remember to use rewards as needed.

**Note:** If you are using the prewritten template, fill in the blanks in the third column with your client at the beginning the exercise.

## Prewritten template

| 1 minute | Outside of the therapy office door | My _____ is going to be hurt or killed. |
| --- | --- | --- |
| 2 minutes | Outside the therapy building | I'll never see _____ again. |
| 5 minutes | In the car | _____ will never come back to get me. |
| 10 minutes | Driving or walking down the street | Bad things are happening to _____. |
| 15 minutes | Caregiver's choice of where to go | Say aloud my worst fear |

## Blank template

|  |  |  |
| --- | --- | --- |
|  |  |  |
|  |  |  |
|  |  |  |
|  |  |  |
|  |  |  |

# Acknowledgments

While I (KSS) had the idea to write this book a few years ago, it wasn't ever something I believed to be possible; and it wouldn't have been possible without the support of many people. A big thank you to all my graduate school (and beyond) mentors who encouraged and inspired me to think outside the box with exposures and get creative with the treatment of my patients. A special thank you to my parents, Paul and Darlene, who inspired my love of reading, learning, and helping others, all of which led to the development of this book. I would also like to thank my husband, Mike, for being incredibly supportive during this journey.

David and I would like to extend our thanks to all those who contributed ideas to our book, including Blaise Worden, Hannah Levy, Kimberly Stevens, and Carolyn Davies. Most of all, we would like to acknowledge our entire team at New Harbinger with a special thanks to our acquisition editor, Tesilya Hanauer, for seeing something special in our book and guiding us through every step of this process.

None of this would be possible without our clients, who have helped us get our creativity flowing to find new ways to help them through exposure. They have been the ones to tell us what has worked and what hasn't and through that have helped us refine our exposure skills. Thank you!

# References

Agras, W. S., Leitenberg, H., Barlow, D. H., Curtis, N. A., Edwards, J., & Wright, D. (1971). Relaxation in systematic desensitization. *Archives of General Psychiatry, 25*(6), 511–514.

Alpers, G. W., & Sell, R. (2008). And yet they correlate: Psychophysiological activation predicts self-report outcomes of exposure therapy in claustrophobia. *Journal of Anxiety Disorders, 22*(7), 1101–1109. doi:10.1016/j.janxdis.2007.11.009

American Psychiatric Association. (2000). *Diagnostic and statistical manual of mental disorders* (4th ed., Text Revision). Washington, DC: American Psychiatric Association.

American Psychiatric Association. (2013). *Diagnostic and statistical manual of mental disorders* (5th ed.). Washington, DC: Author.

Baker, A., Mystkowski, J., Culver, N., Yi, R., Mortazavi, A., & Craske, M. G. (2010). Does habituation matter? Emotional processing theory and exposure therapy for acrophobia. *Behaviour Research and Therapy, 48*(11), 1139–1143. doi:10.1016/j.brat.2010.07.009

Barlow, D. H., Gorman, J. M., Shear, M. K., & Woods, S. W. (2000). Cognitive-behavioral therapy, imipramine, or their combination for panic disorder: A randomized controlled trial. *Journal of The American Medical Association, 283*(19), 2529–2536.

Beard, C., Weisberg, R. B., & Keller, M. B. (2010). Health-related Quality of Life across the anxiety disorders: findings from a sample of primary care patients. *Journal of Anxiety Disorders, 24*(6), 559–564. doi:10.1016/j.janxdis.2010.03.015

Beck, A. T., Emery, G., & Greenberg, R. L. (1985). *Anxiety disorders and phobias: A cognitive perspective.* New York: Basic Books.

Beck, J. G., Gudmundsdottir, B., Palyo, S. A., Miller, L. M., & Grant, D. M. (2006). Rebound effects following deliberate thought suppression: Does PTSD make a difference? *Behavior Therapy, 37*(2), 170–180. doi:10.1016/j.beth.2005.11.002

Becker, C. B., Darius, E., & Schaumberg, K. (2007). An analog study of patient preferences for exposure versus alternative treatments for posttraumatic stress disorder. *Behaviour Research and Therapy, 45*(12), 2861–2873. doi:10.1016/j.brat.2007.05.006

Becker, C. B., Zayfert, C., & Anderson, E. (2004). A survey of psychologists' attitudes towards and utilization of exposure therapy for PTSD. *Behaviour Research and Therapy, 42*(3), 277–292.

Berenz, E. C., Rowe, L., Schumacher, J. A., Stasiewicz, P. R., & Coffey, S. F. (2012). Prolonged exposure therapy for posttraumatic stress disorder among individuals in a residential substance use treatment program: A case series. *Professional Psychology: Research and Practice, 43*(2), 154–161.

Berman, D. E., & Dudai, Y. (2001). Memory extinction, learning anew, and learning the new: Dissociations in the molecular machinery of learning in cortex. *Science, 291*(5512), 2417–2419. doi:10.1126/science.1058165

Bisson, J. I. (2003). Single-session early psychological interventions following traumatic events. *Clinical Psychology Review, 23*(3), 481–499.

Black, D. W., Gaffney, G., Schlosser, S., & Gabel, J. (1998). The impact of obsessive-compulsive disorder on the family: Preliminary findings. *Journal of Nervous and Mental Disease, 186*(7), 440–442.

Bouton, M. E. (1993). Context, time, and memory retrieval in the interference paradigms of Pavlovian learning. *Psychological Bulletin, 114*(1), 80–99.

Brady, K. T., Dansky, B. S., Back, S. E., Foa, E. B., & Carroll, K. M. (2001). Exposure therapy in the treatment of PTSD among cocaine-dependent individuals: Preliminary findings. *Journal of Substance Abuse Treatment, 21*(1), 47–54.

Breslau, N., Kessler, R. C., Chilcoat, H. D., Schultz, L. R., Davis, G. C., & Andreski, P. (1998). Trauma and posttraumatic stress disorder in the community: The 1996 Detroit Area Survey of Trauma. *Archives of General Psychiatry, 55*(7), 626–632.

Bruce, S. L., Ching, T. H. W., & Williams, M. T. (2018). Pedophilia-themed obsessive-compulsive disorder: Assessment, differential diagnosis, and treatment with exposure and response prevention. *Archives of Sexual Behavior, 47*(2), 389–402. doi:10.1007/s10508-017-1031-4

Bryant, R. A., Harvey, A. G., Dang, S. T., Sackville, T., & Basten, C. (1998). Treatment of acute stress disorder: A comparison of cognitive-behavioral therapy and supportive counseling. *Journal of Consulting and Clinical Psychology, 66*(5), 862–866.

Bryant, R. A., Mastrodomenico, J., Hopwood, S., Kenny, L., Cahill, C., Kandris, E., & Taylor, K. (2013). Augmenting cognitive behaviour therapy for post-traumatic stress disorder with emotion tolerance training: A randomized controlled trial. *Psychological Medicine, 43*(10), 2153–2160. doi:10.1017/S0033291713000068

Cain, C. K., Blouin, A. M., & Barad, M. (2003). Temporally massed CS presentations generate more fear extinction than spaced presentations. *Journal of Experimental Psychology: Animal Behavior Processes, 29*(4), 323–333.

Calvocoressi, L., Lewis, B., Harris, M., Trufan, S. J., Goodman, W. K., McDougle, C. J., & Price, L. H. (1995). Family accommodation in obsessive-compulsive disorder. *American Journal of Psychiatry, 152*(3), 441–443.

Chaplin, E. W., & Levine, B. A. (1981). The effects of total exposure duration and inter-rupted versus continuous exposure in flooding therapy. *Behavior Therapy, 12*, 360–368.

Clark, D. M. (1986). A cognitive approach to panic. *Behaviour Research and Therapy, 24*(4), 461–470. doi:10.1016/0005-7967(86)90011-2

Cloitre, M., Courtois, C. A., Charuvastra, A., Carapezza, R., Stolbach, B. C., & Green, B. L. (2011). Treatment of complex PTSD: Results of the ISTSS expert clinician survey on best practices. *Journal of Traumatic Stress, 24*(6), 615–627. doi:10.1002/jts .20697

Cloitre, M., Stolbach, B. C., Herman, J. L., van der Kolk, B., Pynoos, R., Wang, J., & Petkova, E. (2009). A developmental approach to complex PTSD: Childhood and adult cumulative trauma as predictors of symptom complexity. *Journal of Traumatic Stress, 22*(5), 399–408. doi:10.1002/jts.20444

Cloitre, M., Stovall-McClough, K. C., Nooner, K., Zorbas, P., Cherry, S., Jackson, C. L., . . . Petkova, E. (2010). Treatment for PTSD related to childhood abuse: A randomized controlled trial. *American Journal of Psychiatry, 167*(8), 915–924. doi:10.1176/appi.ajp .2010.09081247

Coles, M. E., Frost, R. O., Heimberg, R. G., & Rhéaume, J. (2003). "Not just right experiences": perfectionism, obsessive-compulsive features and general psychopathology. *Behaviour Research and Therapy, 41*(6), 681–700.

Comer, J. S., Blanco, C., Hasin, D. S., Liu, S., Grant, B. F., Turner, J. B., & Olfson, M. (2011). Health-related quality of life across anxiety disorders: Results from the National Epidemiologic Survey on Alcohol and Related Conditions (NESARC). *Journal of Clinical Psychiatry, 72*, 43–50. doi:10.4088/JCP.09m05094blu

Cooper, M. (1996). Obsessive-compulsive disorder: effects on family members. *American Journal of Orthopsychiatry, 66*(2), 296–304.

Craske, M. G., & Barlow, D. H. (2006). *Mastery of your anxiety and panic: Therapist guide* (4th ed.). New York: Oxford University Press.

Craske, M. G., Kircanski, K., Zelikowsky, M., Mystkowski, J., Chowdhury, N., & Baker, A. (2008). Optimizing inhibitory learning during exposure therapy. *Behaviour Research and Therapy, 46*(1), 5–27. doi:10.1016/j.brat.2007.10.003

Craske, M. G., Treanor, M., Conway, C. C., Zbozinek, T., & Vervliet, B. (2014). Maximizing exposure therapy: An inhibitory learning approach. *Behaviour Research and Therapy, 58*, 10–23. doi:10.1016/j.brat.2014.04.006

Davey, G. (1993). Factors influencing self-rated fear to a novel animal. *Cognition and Emotion, 7*, 461–471.

Deacon, B. J., Kemp, J. J., Dixon, L. J., Sy, J. T., Farrell, N. R., & Zhang, A. R. (2013). Maximizing the efficacy of interoceptive exposure by optimizing inhibitory learning: A randomized controlled trial. *Behaviour Research and Therapy, 51*(9), 588–596. doi:10.1016/j.brat.2013.06.006

Deacon, B. J., Lickel, J. J., Farrell, N. R., Kemp, J. J., & Hipol, L. J. (2013). Therapist perceptions and delivery of interoceptive exposure for panic disorder. *Journal of Anxiety Disorders, 27*(2), 259–264. doi:10.1016/j.janxdis.2013.02.004

Deacon, B. J., Sy, J. T., Lickel, J. J., & Nelson, E. A. (2010). Does the judicious use of safety behaviors improve the efficacy and acceptability of exposure therapy for claustrophobic fear? *Journal of Behavior Therapy and Experimental Psychiatry, 41*(1), 71–80. doi:10.1016/j.jbtep.2009.10.004

de Jong, P. J., Andrea, H., & Muris, P. (1997). Spider phobia in children: Disgust and fear before and after treatment. *Behaviour Research and Therapy, 35*(6), 559–562.

Delgado, M. R., Nearing, K. I., Ledoux, J. E., & Phelps, E. A. (2008). Neural circuitry underlying the regulation of conditioned fear and its relation to extinction. *Neuron, 59*(5), 829–838. doi:10.1016/j.neuron.2008.06.029

DuPont, R. L., Rice, D. P., Miller, L. S., Shiraki, S. S., Rowland, C. R., & Harwood, H. J. (1996). Economic costs of anxiety disorders. *Anxiety, 2*(4), 167–172.

Faravelli, C., Salvatori, S., Galassi, F., Aiazzi, L., Drei, C., & Cabras, P. (1997). Epidemiology of somatoform disorders: a community survey in Florence. *Social Psychiatry and Psychiatric Epidemiology, 32*(1), 24–29.

Foa, E. B., & Kozak, M. J. (1986). Emotional processing of fear: Exposure to corrective information. *Psychological Bulletin, 99*(1), 20–35. doi:10.1037/0033-2909.99.1.20

Foa, E. B., Kozak, M. J., Goodman, W. K., Hollander, E., Jenike, M. A., & Rasmussen, S. A. (1995). DSM-IV field trial: Obsessive-compulsive disorder. *American Journal of Psychiatry, 152*(1), 90–96.

Foa, E. B., Liebowitz, M. R., Kozak, M. J., Davies, S., Campeas, R., Franklin, M. E., . . . Tu, X. (2005). Randomized, placebo-controlled trial of exposure and ritual prevention, clomipramine, and their combination in the treatment of obsessive-compulsive disorder. *American Journal of Psychiatry, 162*(1), 151–161. doi:10.1176/appi.ajp.162.1.151

Foa, E. B., Riggs, D. S., Massie, E. D., & Yarczower, M. (1995). The impact of fear activation and anger on the efficacy of exposure treatment for posttraumatic stress disorder. *Behavior Therapy, 26*, 487–499.

Foa, E. B., Zoellner, L. A., Feeny, N. C., Hembree, E. A., & Alvarez-Conrad, J. (2002). Does imaginal exposure exacerbate PTSD symptoms? *Journal of Consulting and Clinical Psychology, 70*(4), 1022–1028.

Franklin, M. E., Kratz, H. E., Freeman, J. B., Ivarsson, T., Heyman, I., Sookman, D., . . . Accreditation Task Force of The Canadian Institute for Obsessive Compulsive, D. (2015). Cognitive-behavioral therapy for pediatric obsessive-compulsive disorder: Empirical review and clinical recommendations. *Psychiatry Research, 227*(1), 78–92. doi:10.1016/j.psychres.2015.02.009

Gilboa-Schechtman, E., Foa, E. B., Shafran, N., Aderka, I. M., Powers, M. B., Rachamim, L., . . . Apter, A. (2010). Prolonged exposure versus dynamic therapy for adolescent

PTSD: A pilot randomized controlled trial. *Journal of the American Academy of Child and Adolescent Psychiatry, 49*(10), 1034–1042. doi:10.1016/j.jaac.2010.07.014

Goisman, R. M., Rogers, M. P., Steketee, G. S., Warshaw, M. G., Cuneo, P., & Keller, M. B. (1993). Utilization of behavioral methods in a multicenter anxiety disorders study. *Journal of Clinical Psychiatry, 54*(6), 213–218.

Goldstein, A. J., & Chambless, D. L. (1978). A reanalysis of agoraphobia. *Behavior Therapy, 9*, 47–59.

Grant, B. F., Hasin, D. S., Stinson, F. S., Dawson, D. A., Goldstein, R. B., Smith, S., . . . Saha, T. D. (2006). The epidemiology of DSM-IV panic disorder and agoraphobia in the United States: Results from the National Epidemiologic Survey on Alcohol and Related Conditions. *Journal of Clinical Psychiatry, 67*(3), 363–374.

Grayson, J. B., Foa, E. B., & Steketee, G. (1982). Habituation during exposure treatment: Distraction vs attention-focusing. *Behaviour Research and Therapy, 20*(4), 323–328.

Hans, E., & Hiller, W. (2013). A meta-analysis of nonrandomized effectiveness studies on outpatient cognitive behavioral therapy for adult anxiety disorders. *Clinical Psychology Review, 33*(8), 954–964. doi:10.1016/j.cpr.2013.07.003

Hedtke, K. A., Kendall, P. C., & Tiwari, S. (2009). Safety-seeking and coping behavior during exposure tasks with anxious youth. *Journal of Clinical Child and Adolescent Psychology, 38*(1), 1–15. doi:10.1080/15374410802581055

Heimberg, R. G., Liebowitz, M. R., Hope, D. A., Schneier, F. R., Holt, C. S., Welkowitz, L. A., . . . Klein, D. F. (1998). Cognitive behavioral group therapy versus phenelzine therapy for social phobia: 12-week outcome. *Archives of General Psychiatry, 55*(12), 1133–1141.

Hembree, E. A., Foa, E. B., Dorfan, N. M., Street, G. P., Kowalski, J., & Tu, X. (2003). Do patients drop out prematurely from exposure therapy for PTSD? *Journal of Traumatic Stress, 16*(6), 555–562. doi:10.1023/B:JOTS.0000004078.93012.7d

Hofmann, S. G., & Smits, J. A. (2008). Cognitive-behavioral therapy for adult anxiety disorders: A meta-analysis of randomized placebo-controlled trials. *Journal of Clinical Psychiatry, 69*(4), 621–632.

Institute of Medicine. (2008). *Treatment of posttraumatic stress disorder: An assessment of the evidence.* Washington, DC: National Academies Press.

Jonas, D. E., Cusack, K., Forneris, C. A., Wilkins, T. M., Sonis, J., Middleton, J. C., . . . Gaynes, B. N. (2013). *Psychological and pharmacological treatments for adults with posttraumatic stress disorder (PTSD): Comparative effectiveness review No. 92.* Agency for Healthcare Research and Quality.

Jordan, B. K., Marmar, C. R., Fairbank, J. A., Schlenger, W. E., Kulka, R. A., Hough, R. L., & Weiss, D. S. (1992). Problems in families of male Vietnam veterans with posttraumatic stress disorder. *Journal of Consulting and Clinical Psychology, 60*(6), 916–926.

Kalra, H., Kamath, P., Trivedi, J. K., & Janca, A. (2008). Caregiver burden in anxiety disorders. *Current Opinion in Psychiatry, 21*(1), 70–73.

Kamphuis, J. H., & Telch, M. J. (2000). Effects of distraction and guided threat reappraisal on fear reduction during exposure-based treatments for specific fears. *Behaviour Research and Therapy, 38*(12), 1163–1181.

Kendall, P. C., Robin, J. A., Hedtke, K. A., Suveg, C., Flannery-Schroeder, E., & Gosch, E. (2006). Considering CBT with anxious youth? Think exposures. *Cognitive and Behavioral Practice, 12*(1), 136–148.

Kessler, R. C., Chiu, W. T., Jin, R., Ruscio, A. M., Shear, K., & Walters, E. E. (2006). The epidemiology of panic attacks, panic disorder, and agoraphobia in the National Comorbidity Survey Replication. *Archives of General Psychiatry, 63*(4), 415–424. doi:10.1001/archpsyc.63.4.415

Kessler, R. C., Petukhova, M., Sampson, N. A., Zaslavsky, A. M., & Wittchen, H. U. (2012). Twelve-month and lifetime prevalence and lifetime morbid risk of anxiety and mood disorders in the United States. *International Journal of Methods in Psychiatric Research, 21*(3), 169–184.

Kessler, R. C., Sonnega, A., Bromet, E., Hughes, M., & Nelson, C. B. (1995). Posttraumatic stress disorder in the National Comorbidity Survey. *Archives of General Psychiatry, 52*(12), 1048–1060. doi:10.1001/archpsyc.1995.03950240066012

Kim, E. J. (2005). The effect of the decreased safety behaviors on anxiety and negative thoughts in social phobics. *Journal of Anxiety Disorders, 19*(1), 69–86. doi:10.1016/j.janxdis.2003.11.002

Kozak, M. J., & Montgomery, G. K. (1981). Multimodal behavioral treatment of recurrent injury-scene-elicited fainting (vasodepressor syncope). *Behavioural Psychotherapy,* 316–321.

Leonard, H. L., & Swedo, S. E. (2001). Paediatric autoimmune neuropsychiatric disorders associated with streptococcal infection (PANDAS). *International Journal of Neuropsychopharmacology, 4*(2), 191–198. doi:10.1017/S1461145701002371

Lebowitz, E. R. (2013). Parent-based treatment for childhood and adolescent OCD. *Journal of Obsessive-Compulsive and Related Disorders, 2*(4), 425–431.

Lebowitz, E. R., Omer, H., Hermes, H., & Scahill, L. (2014). Parent training for childhood anxiety disorders: The SPACE program. *Cognitive and Behavioral Practice, 21*(4), 456–469.

Levenson, R. W. (1992). Autonomic nervous system differences among emotions. *Psychological Science, 3,* 23–27.

Levy, H. C., & Radomsky, A. S. (2014). Safety behaviour enhances the acceptability of exposure. *Cognitive Behaviour Therapy, 43*(1), 83–92. doi:10.1080/16506073.2013.819376

Lewin, A. B., Park, J. M., Jones, A. M., Crawford, E. A., De Nadai, A. S., Menzel, J., . . . Storch, E. A. (2014). Family-based exposure and response prevention therapy for preschool-aged children with obsessive-compulsive disorder: A pilot randomized controlled trial. *Behaviour Research and Therapy, 56*, 30–38. doi:10.1016/j.brat.2014.02.001

Linehan, M. M. (2014). *DBT Skills Training Manual.* New York: The Guilford Press.

Lochner, C., Mogotsi, M., du Toit, P. L., Kaminer, D., Niehaus, D. J., & Stein, D. J. (2003). Quality of life in anxiety disorders: A comparison of obsessive-compulsive disorder, social anxiety disorder, and panic disorder. *Psychopathology, 36*, 255–262.

Looper, K. J., & Kirmayer, L. J. (2001). Hypochondriacal concerns in a community population. *Psychological Medicine, 31*(4), 577–584.

MacLeod, C., Mathews, A., & Tata, P. (1986). Attentional bias in emotional disorders. *Journal of Abnormal Psychology, 95*(1), 15–20.

March, J. S., & Mulle, K. (1998). *OCD in children and adolescents: A cognitive-behavioral treatment manual.* New York: Guilford Press.

McKay, D. (2006). Treating disgust reactions in contamination-based obsessive-compulsive disorder. *Journal of Behavior Therapy and Experimental Psychiatry, 37*(1), 53–59.

Merckelbach, H., de Jong, P. J., Arntz, A., & Schouten, E. (1993). The role of evaluative learning and disgust sensitivity in the etiology and treatment of spider phobia. *Advances in Behavior Research and Therapy, 15*, 243–255.

Meuret, A. E., Seidel, A., Rosenfield, B., Hofmann, S. G., & Rosenfield, D. (2012). Does fear reactivity during exposure predict panic symptom reduction? *Journal of Consulting and Clinical Psychology, 80*(5), 773–785. doi:10.1037/a0028032

Miller, W. R., & Rollnick, S. (2013). *Motivational interviewing: Helping people change* (3rd ed.). New York: Guilford Press.

Mills, K. L., Teesson, M., Back, S. E., Brady, K. T., Baker, A. L., Hopwood, S., . . . Ewer, P. L. (2012). Integrated exposure-based therapy for co-occurring posttraumatic stress disorder and substance dependence: A randomized controlled trial. *Journal of The American Medical Association, 308*(7), 690–699.

Mineka, S., Mystkowski, J. L., Hladek, D., & Rodriguez, B. I. (1999). The effects of changing contexts on return of fear following exposure therapy for spider fear. *Journal of Consulting and Clinical Psychology, 67*(4), 599–604.

Nacasch, N., Huppert, J. D., Su, Y. J., Kivity, Y., Dinshtein, Y., Yeh, R., & Foa, E. B. (2015). Are 60-minute prolonged exposure sessions with 20-minute imaginal exposure to traumatic memories sufficient to successfully treat PTSD? A randomized noninferiority clinical trial. *Behavior Therapy, 46*(3), 328–341. doi:10.1016/j.beth.2014.12.002

Nelson, E. A., Deacon, B. J., Lickel, J. J., & Sy, J. T. (2010). Targeting the probability versus cost of feared outcomes in public speaking anxiety. *Behaviour Research and Therapy, 48*(4), 282–289. doi:10.1016/j.brat.2009.11.007

Norton, P. J., & Price, E. C. (2007). A meta-analytic review of adult cognitive-behavioral treatment outcome across the anxiety disorders. *Journal of Nervous and Mental Disease, 195*(6), 521–531. doi:10.1097/01.nmd.0000253843.70149.9a

Olatunji, B. O., Cisler, J. M., & Tolin, D. F. (2007). Quality of life in the anxiety disorders: A meta-analytic review. *Clinical Psychology Review, 27*(5), 572–581. doi:10.1016/j.cpr.2007.01.015

Olatunji, B. O., Smits, J. A., Connolly, K., Willems, J., & Lohr, J. M. (2007). Examination of the decline in fear and disgust during exposure to threat-relevant stimuli in blood-injection-injury phobia. *Journal of Anxiety Disorders, 21*(3), 445–455.

Ollendick, T. H., Ost, L. G., Reuterskiold, L., Costa, N., Cederlund, R., Sirbu, C., . . . Jarrett, M. A. (2009). One-session treatment of specific phobias in youth: A randomized clinical trial in the United States and Sweden. *Journal of Consulting and Clinical Psychology, 77*(3), 504–516. doi:10.1037/a0015158

Öst, L. G. (1989). One-session treatment for specific phobias. *Behaviour Research and Therapy, 27*(1), 1–7.

Öst, L. G., Fellenius, J., & Sterner, U. (1991). Applied tension, exposure in vivo, and tension-only in the treatment of blood phobia. *Behaviour Research and Therapy, 29*(6), 561–574.

Otto, M. W., Simon, N. M., Olatunji, B. O., Sung, S. C., & Pollack, M. H. (2011). *10-minute CBT: Integrating cognitive-behavioral strategies into your practcie.* New York: Oxford University Press.

Parsons, T. D., & Rizzo, A. A. (2008). Affective outcomes of virtual reality exposure therapy for anxiety and specific phobias: A meta-analysis. *Journal of Behavior Therapy and Experimental Psychiatry, 39*(3), 250–261. doi:10.1016/j.jbtep.2007.07.007

Piacentini, J., Bergman, R. L., Chang, S., Langley, A., Peris, T., Wood, J. J., & McCracken, J. (2011). Controlled comparison of family cognitive behavioral therapy and psychoeducation/relaxation training for child obsessive-compulsive disorder. *Journal of the American Academy of Child and Adolescent Psychiatry, 50*(11), 1149–1161. doi:10.1016/j.jaac.2011.08.003

Pincus, D. B., May, J. E., Whitton, S. W., Mattis, S. G., & Barlow, D. H. (2010). Cognitive-behavioral treatment of panic disorder in adolescence. *Journal of Clinical Child and Adolescent Psychology, 39*(5), 638–649. doi:10.1080/15374416.2010.501288

Powers, M. B., & Emmelkamp, P. M. (2008). Virtual reality exposure therapy for anxiety disorders: A meta-analysis. *Journal of Anxiety Disorders, 22*(3), 561–569. doi:10.1016/j.janxdis.2007.04.006

Powers, M. B., Halpern, J. M., Ferenschak, M. P., Gillihan, S. J., & Foa, E. B. (2010). A meta-analytic review of prolonged exposure for posttraumatic stress disorder. *Clinical Psychology Review, 30*(6), 635–641. doi:10.1016/j.cpr.2010.04.007

Powers, M. B., Smits, J. A., & Telch, M. J. (2004). Disentangling the effects of safety-behavior utilization and safety-behavior availability during exposure-based treatment: A placebo-controlled trial. *Journal of Consulting and Clinical Psychology, 72*(3), 448–454. doi:10.1037/0022-006X.72.3.448

Powers, M. B., Smits, J. A., Whitley, D., Bystritsky, A., & Telch, M. J. (2008). The effect of attributional processes concerning medication taking on return of fear. *Journal of Consulting and Clinical Psychology, 76*(3), 478–490. doi:10.1037/0022-006X.76.3.478

Prochaska, J. O., & DiClemente, C. C. (1982). Transtheoretical therapy: Toward a more integrated model of change. *Psychotherapy: Theory, Research, and Practice, 19*, 276–288.

Rachman, S. J., Shafran, R., Radomsky, A. S., & Zysk, E. (2011). Reducing contamination by exposure plus safety behaviour. *Journal of Behavior Therapy and Experimental Psychiatry, 42*(3), 397–404. doi:10.1016/j.jbtep.2011.02.010

Rescorla, R. A. (2006). Deepened extinction from compound stimulus presentation. *Journal of Experimental Psychology: Animal Behavior Processes, 32*(2), 135–144. doi:10.1037/0097-7403.32.2.135

Rescorla, R. A., & Wagner, A. R. (1972). A theory of Pavlovian conditioning: Variations in the effectiveness of reinforcement and nonreinforcement. In R. O. Mowrer & S. Klein (Eds.), *Handbook of contemporary learning theories.* Mahwah, NJ: Lawrence Erlbaum Associates.

Riggs, D. S., Byrne, C. A., Weathers, F. W., & Litz, B. T. (1998). The quality of the intimate relationships of male Vietnam veterans: problems associated with posttraumatic stress disorder. *Journal of Traumatic Stress, 11*(1), 87–101.

Rose, S., Bisson, J., Churchill, R., & Wessely, S. (2001). Psychological debriefing for preventing post traumatic stress disorder (PTSD). *The Cochrane Database of Systematic Reviews*(3), CD000560. doi:10.1002/14651858.CD000560

Rozin, P., & Fallon, A. E. (1987). A perspective on disgust. *Psychological Review, 94*(1), 23–41.

Safran, J. D., Muran, J. C., & Eubanks-Carter, C. (2011). Repairing alliance ruptures. In J. C. Norcross (Ed.), *Psychotherapy relationships that work: Evidence-based responsiveness* (2nd ed., pp. 224–238). New York: Oxford University Press.

Sawchuk, C. N., Lohr, J. M., Tolin, D. F., Lee, T. C., & Kleinknecht, R. A. (2000). Disgust sensitivity and contamination fears in spider and blood-injection-injury phobias. *Behaviour Research and Therapy, 38*(8), 753–762.

Schare, M. L., & Wyatt, K. P. (2013). On the evolving nature of exposure therapy. *Behavior Modification, 37*(2), 243–256. doi:10.1177/0145445513477421

Schmidt, N. B., Woolaway-Bickel, K., Trakowski, J., Santiago, H., Storey, J., Koselka, M., & Cook, J. (2000). Dismantling cognitive-behavioral treatment for panic disorder:

Questioning the utility of breathing retraining. *Journal of Consulting and Clinical Psychology, 68*(3), 417–424.

Sloan, T., & Telch, M. J. (2002). The effects of safety-seeking behavior and guided threat reappraisal on fear reduction during exposure: An experimental investigation. *Behaviour Research and Therapy, 40,* 235–251.

Smits, J. A., Telch, M. J., & Randall, P. K. (2002). An examination of the decline in fear and disgust during exposure–based treatment. *Behaviour Research and Therapy, 40*(11), 1243-1253.

Solomon, R. L., Kamin, L. J., & Wynne, L. C. (1953). Traumatic avoidance learning: The outcomes of several extinction procedures with dogs. *Journal of Abnormal Psychology, 48*(2), 291–302.

Stewart, R. E., & Chambless, D. L. (2009). Cognitive-behavioral therapy for adult anxiety disorders in clinical practice: A meta-analysis of effectiveness studies. *Journal of Consulting and Clinical Psychology, 77*(4), 595–606. doi:10.1037/a0016032

Stone, M., & Borkovec, T. D. (1975). The paradoxical effect of brief CS exposure on analogue phobic subjects. *Behaviour Research and Therapy, 13*(1), 51–54.

Swedo, S. E., Leckman, J. F., & Rose, N. R. (2012). From research subgroup to clinical syndrome: Modifying the PANDAS criteria to describe PANS (pediatric acute-onset neuropsychiatric syndrome). *Pediatric Therapeutics, 2*(2), 113.

Telch, M. J., Valentiner, D. P., Ilai, D., Young, P. R., Powers, M. B., & Smits, J. A. (2004). Fear activation and distraction during the emotional processing of claustrophobic fear. *Journal of Behavior Therapy and Experimental Psychiatry, 35*(3), 219–232. doi:10.1016/j.jbtep.2004.03.004

Tolin, D. F. (2016). *Doing CBT: A comprehensive guide to working with behaviors, thoughts, and emotions.* New York: Guilford Press.

Tolin, D. F., Abramowitz, J. S., Przeworski, A., & Foa, E. B. (2002). Thought suppression in obsessive-compulsive disorder. *Behaviour Research and Therapy, 40*(11), 1255–1274.

van Emmerik, A. A., Kamphuis, J. H., Hulsbosch, A. M., & Emmelkamp, P. M. (2002). Single session debriefing after psychological trauma: A meta-analysis. *Lancet, 360*(9335), 766–771. doi:10.1016/S0140-6736(02)09897-5

van Minnen, A., & Hagenaars, M. (2002). Fear activation and habituation patterns as early process predictors of response to prolonged exposure treatment in PTSD. *Journal of Traumatic Stress, 15*(5), 359–367.

Van Noppen, B. L., & Steketee, G. (2003). Family responses and multifamily behavioral treatment for obsessive-compulsive disorder. *Brief Treatment and Crisis Intervention, 3,* 231–247.

Vansteenwegen, D., Vervliet, B., Iberico, C., Baeyens, F., Van den Bergh, O., & Hermans, D. (2007). The repeated confrontation with videotapes of spiders in multiple contexts attenuates renewal of fear in spider-anxious students. *Behaviour Research and Therapy, 45*(6), 1169–1179.

Veale, D., Freeston, M., Krebs, G., Heyman, I., & Salkovskis, P. (2009). Risk assessment and management in obsessive-compulsive disorder. *Advances in Psychiatric Treatment, 15*, 332–343.

Vella-Zarb, R. A., Cohen, J. N., McCabe, R. E., & Rowa, K. (2017). Differentiating sexual thoughts in obsessive-compulsive disorder from paraphilias and nonparaphilic sexual disorders. *Cognitive and Behavioral Practice, 24*, 342–352.

Veltro, F., Magliano, L., Lobrace, S., Morosini, P. L., & Maj, M. (1994). Burden on key relatives of patients with schizophrenia vs neurotic disorders: A pilot study. *Social Psychiatry and Psychiatric Epidemiology, 29*(2), 66–70.

Verbosky, S. J., & Ryan, D. A. (1988). Female partners of Vietnam veterans: Stress by proximity. *Issues in Mental Health Nursing, 9*(1), 95–104.

Wegner, D. M., Schneider, D. J., Carter, S. R., & White, T. L. (1987). Paradoxical effects of thought suppression. *Journal of Personality and Social Psychology, 53*, 5–13.

Weisman, J. S., & Rodebaugh, T. L. (2018). Exposure therapy augmentation: A review and extension of techniques informed by an inhibitory learning approach. *Clinical Psychology Review, 59*, 41–51. doi:10.1016/j.cpr.2017.10.010

Westra, H. A., Stewart, S. H., & Conrad, B. E. (2002). Naturalistic manner of benzodiazepine use and cognitive behavioral therapy outcome in panic disorder with agoraphobia. *Journal of Anxiety Disorders, 16*(3), 233–246.

Wolitzky, K. B., & Telch, M. J. (2009). Augmenting in vivo exposure with fear antagonistic actions: A preliminary test. *Behavior Therapy, 40*(1), 57–71. doi:10.1016/j.beth .2007.12.006

Wolpe, J. (1961). The systematic desensitization treatment of neuroses. *Journal of Nervous and Mental Disease, 132*, 189–203.

Wolpe, J. (1990). *The practice of behavior therapy* (4th ed.). New York: Pergamon Press.

Woods, A. M., & Bouton, M. E. (2007). Occasional reinforced responses during extinction can slow the rate of reacquisition of an operant response. *Learning and Motivation, 38*(1), 56–74. doi:10.1016/j.lmot.2006.07.003

World Health Organization. (2010). *WHO guidelines on drawing blood: Best practices in phlebotomy.* Geneva, Switzerland: Author.

Xue, C., Ge, Y., Tang, B., Liu, Y., Kang, P., Wang, M., & Zhang, L. (2015). A meta-analysis of risk factors for combat-related PTSD among military personnel and veterans. *PLoS One, 10*(3), e0120270. doi:10.1371/journal.pone.0120270

Zoellner, L. A., Feeny, N. C., Cochran, B., & Pruitt, L. (2003). Treatment choice for PTSD. *Behaviour Research and Therapy, 41*(8), 879–886.

**Kristen S. Springer, PhD**, is a licensed clinical psychologist in Massachusetts with a private practice in the greater Boston, MA, area. She earned her doctoral degree from the University of Florida, and completed her postdoctoral clinical and research training at the Anxiety Disorders Center and the Center for Cognitive Behavioral Therapy at the Hartford Hospital Institute of Living in Hartford, CT. She continued working at the Anxiety Disorders Center as a staff psychologist before opening her private practice where she specializes in the assessment and treatment of obsessive-compulsive disorder (OCD) and anxiety disorders in adolescents and adults. Springer has authored several book chapters and scientific journal articles in the fields of anxiety, hoarding, OCD, and chronic pain. You can learn more about her at www.massanxietytreatment.com.

**David F. Tolin, PhD**, is founder and director of the Anxiety Disorders Center and the Center for Cognitive Behavioral Therapy at the Hartford Hospital Institute of Living in Hartford, CT. He is adjunct professor of psychiatry at Yale University School of Medicine, and maintains a private practice in the greater Hartford area. Tolin has authored more than 150 scientific journal articles, as well as the books, *Face Your Fears* and *Doing CBT*.

# Index

# Real change *is* possible

For more than forty-five years, New Harbinger has published proven-effective self-help books and pioneering workbooks to help readers of all ages and backgrounds improve mental health and well-being, and achieve lasting personal growth. In addition, our spirituality books offer profound guidance for deepening awareness and cultivating healing, self-discovery, and fulfillment.

Founded by psychologist Matthew McKay and Patrick Fanning, New Harbinger is proud to be an independent, employee-owned company. Our books reflect our core values of integrity, innovation, commitment, sustainability, compassion, and trust. Written by leaders in the field and recommended by therapists worldwide, New Harbinger books are practical, accessible, and provide real tools for real change.

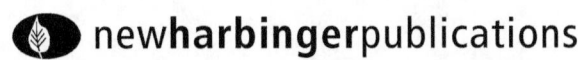 **newharbinger**publications

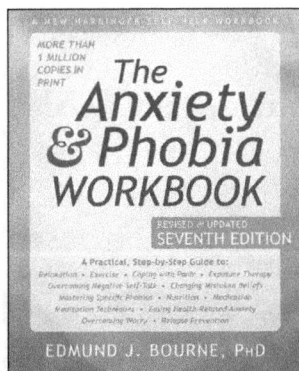
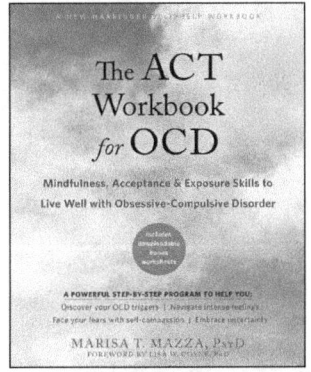
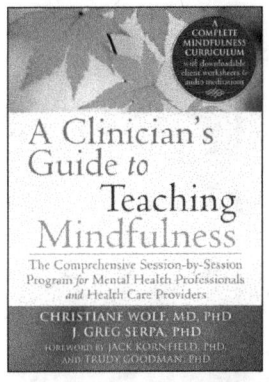
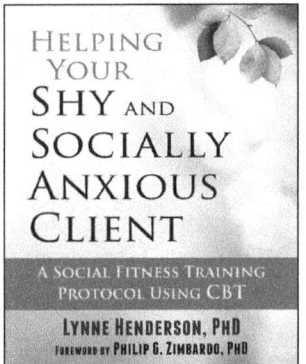
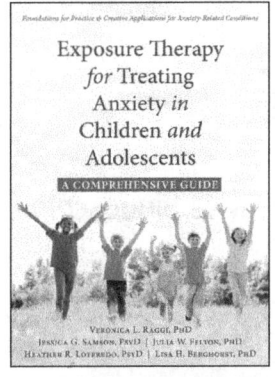
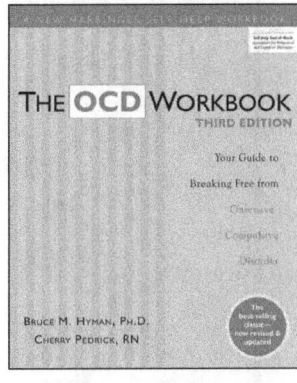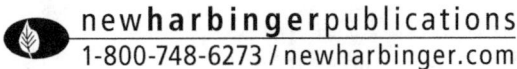

Register your **new harbinger** titles for additional benefits!

When you register your **new harbinger** title—purchased in any format, from any source—you get access to benefits like the following:

- Downloadable accessories like printable worksheets and extra content

- Instructional videos and audio files

- Information about updates, corrections, and new editions

Not every title has accessories, but we're adding new material all the time.

Access free accessories in 3 easy steps:

1. Sign in at NewHarbinger.com (or **register** to create an account).

2. Click on **register a book**. Search for your title and click the **register** button when it appears.

3. Click on the **book cover or title** to go to its details page. Click on **accessories** to view and access files.

That's all there is to it!

If you need help, visit:

NewHarbinger.com/accessories

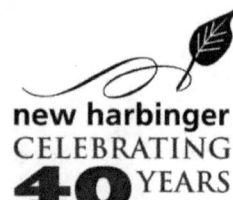

**new harbinger**
CELEBRATING
**40** YEARS